Advance Praise for
Understanding Your Migraines

"Finally, a book that takes years of clinical experience and decades of scientific discoveries and boils them down into simple, easy-to-understand language, giving patients insight they can use to manage their headaches successfully. *Understanding Your Migraines* gives hope to the most challenging-to-treat headache sufferers. A true testimony to the power of academic medicine, this book reflects the many thousands of hours the authors spent listening to their patients, addressing their concerns, taking endless notes, making symptom-based diagnoses, practicing evidence-based medicine, treating the patients themselves rather than their lab tests and images, ensuring the benefits of treatments, not blaming the patient when treatments fail, and most importantly, taking the time to educate patients about their illnesses."

—**Rami Burstein, PhD**, John Hedley-Whyte Professor of Anaesthesia and Neuroscience, Harvard Medical School and Beth Israel Deaconess Medical Center, Boston, MA

"*Understanding Your Migraines*, written by two pre-eminent thought leaders in the headache field, is a comprehensive look at migraine and other related disorders. Each of the chapters begins with a case history to introduce a topic and as the information is delivered the authors refer to the case to drive home their point. While we headache medicine specialists discuss these issues with our patients, not all clinicians have the time or the expertise required. This book is useful in that it reinforces what we clinicians tell our patients but also provides education on topics that may not have not been broached during the visit."

—**Lawrence C. Newman, MD**, Director, The Headache Institute, Mount Sinai St. Luke's, New York, NY

"Migraine is a common, disabling, and often misunderstood disease. For those contending with migraine, it is a challenge to find current and reliable information on what migraine is, and what it isn't, and what measures will bring it under control. *Understanding Your Migraines* now provides welcome and authoritative guidance from two renowned migraine doctors and researchers. Written in an engaging and clear style, which is punctuated by illustrative patient vignettes, Professors Levin and Ward logically guide the reader to understand the process of diagnosing migraine and the multiple approaches to effective migraine therapy."

—**Robert E. Shapiro, MD, PhD**, Professor of Neurological Sciences, Larner College of Medicine, University of Vermont, Burlington, VT

UNDERSTANDING YOUR MIGRAINES

Understanding Your Migraines

A Guide for Patients and Families

Morris Levin, MD

Professor of Neurology
Director, Headache Center
University of California at San Francisco
San Francisco, CA

Thomas N. Ward, MD

Professor of Neurology, Emeritus
Geisel School of Medicine at Dartmouth
Hanover, NH

OXFORD
UNIVERSITY PRESS

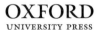

OXFORD
UNIVERSITY PRESS

Oxford University Press is a department of the University of Oxford. It furthers
the University's objective of excellence in research, scholarship, and education
by publishing worldwide. Oxford is a registered trade mark of Oxford University
Press in the UK and certain other countries.

Published in the United States of America by Oxford University Press
198 Madison Avenue, New York, NY 10016, United States of America.

Library of Congress Cataloging-in-Publication Data
Names: Levin, Morris, 1955– author. | Ward, Thomas N., author.
Title: Understanding your migraines : a guide for patients and families / by Morris
Levin, MD, Director, Headache Center, Department of Neurology, University of
California at San Francisco, San Francisco, CA, Thomas N. Ward, MD, Professor of
Neurology, Emeritus, Geisel School of Medicine at Dartmouth, Hanover, NH.
Description: New York, NY : Oxford University Press, [2017] | Includes index.
Identifiers: LCCN 2016039465 | ISBN 9780190209155 (alk. paper)
Subjects: LCSH: Migraine—Popular works. | Migraine—Case studies.
Classification: LCC RC392.L45 2017 | DDC 616.8/4912—dc23
LC record available at https://lccn.loc.gov/2016039465

1 3 5 7 9 8 6 4 2

Printed by Sheridan Books, Inc., United States of America

I would like to dedicate this book to my patients. They are the ones who bear the burden of migraine, usually with great courage and resilience. They have helped me grow as a physician and headache specialist, and I am grateful for their patience with that process. I also dedicate it to my wife, Karen, for putting up with my spending so much time with this project.

M. L.

I dedicate this book to the headache patients I have worked with over the years and to their families who share the burden with them.

T. N. W.

CONTENTS

Preface | xv

1. What Type of Headache Do I Have? | 1
   Primary Headaches | 2
      Migraine | 2
      Tension-Type Headaches | 4
      Cluster Headaches | 6
      Rare Primary Headache Conditions | 7
   Secondary Headaches | 8
      Post-traumatic Headaches | 9
      Blood Vessels and Headaches | 10
      Intracranial Hypertension Headaches | 12
      Low Intracranial Pressure Headaches | 12
      Brain Malformations | 12
      Brain Tumors | 13
      Seizures and Headaches | 13
      Medication Overuse Headaches | 13
      Recreational Drug Use and Headaches | 16
      Medical Illness and Headaches | 17
      Mental Illness and Headaches | 17

Neuralgia | 18

Summary | 18

2. Do I Have Migraine? | 21

    What Is Migraine? | 24

    Migraine Triggers | 26

    Migraine Aura | 29

    Migraine Features | 29

    The Aftermath of a Migraine Attack | 30

    Medical Conditions Associated with Migraine | 30

    Diagnosing Migraine: Our Examples | 32

3. The Nature and Causes of Migraine | 35

    Migraine in History | 36

    Scientific Advances in Understanding Migraine | 37

    Aura | 37

    Genetics | 41

4. The Impact of Migraine | 43

    Disability Due to Migraine | 45

    Goals in Managing Migraine | 47

    Some Practical Examples | 50

5. Relieving a Migraine Headache: The Best Medical
    Treatments | 53

    Tailoring Treatment | 54

    The Fundamentals | 55

    Choosing Treatment Options Based on Characteristics of
       Attacks | 56

    Options for Recurrence and Rescue | 59

    Successful Migraine Relief: Our Examples | 61

6. Relieving a Migraine Headache: Non-medicinal
   Approaches | 65

   Acting on Warnings of an Impending Attack | 66

   Simple Physical Measures | 67

   Caffeine, Aromatherapy, and Herbal Approaches | 67

   Behavioral Medicine Techniques | 70

7. Preventing Migraine: Medical Choices | 71

   How to Choose Preventive Medication | 71

   Options for Preventive Medication | 75

      Beta Blockers | 77

      Antidepressants | 77

      Anti-seizure Medications | 78

      Other Preventives | 79

   Caution Regarding Pregnancy | 80

   Successful Medicinal Migraine Prevention: Our Examples | 81

8. Preventing Migraine: Non-medicinal and Alternative
   Approaches | 83

   Herbal Treatments | 84

   Physical Exercise | 86

   Manual Techniques | 86

   Nutritional Intervention | 87

   Dietary Supplements | 89

   Meditation and Relaxation Approaches | 89

   Successful Non-medicinal Migraine Prevention: An
      Example | 92

9. Migraine in Children and Adolescents | 95

   Distinctive Aspects of Childhood Migraine | 95

   Prevention and Treatment | 97

   Managing the Impact of Childhood Migraine | 100

10. Migraine During Pregnancy and When Breastfeeding | 103

Three Phases of Migraine Management Surrounding
Pregnancy | 105
Before Pregnancy | 105
During Pregnancy | 105
After Delivery | 106

Medication Use and Risks | 106

Treating Migraines While Breastfeeding | 110

Migraine in Pregnancy: Some Successful Examples | 111

11. Chronic Migraine | 113

How Chronic Migraine Develops | 116

Treatment and Management | 118

Successfully Managing Chronic Migraine: Some
Examples | 122

12. Newer and Experimental Treatments for Migraine and
Other Headaches | 125

New Forms of Medication | 126

Nerve Blocks | 127

Nerve Stimulation | 129

Magnetic Stimulation | 131

Infusions and Hospital Treatment | 131

Progress and Patience | 133

13. Tension-Type Headache: The "Usual" Headache | 135

What Is Tension-Type Headache? | 135

Mimics of Tension-Type Headache | 137

Treating Tension-Type Headache | 139

Successfully Managing Tension-Type Headache: An
Example | 140

14. Unusual Headaches: Cluster Headache, Other Trigeminal Autonomic Cephalalgias, and New Daily Persistent Headache | 143

Trigeminal Autonomic Cephalalgias: Cluster Headache and Its Relatives | 144
    Cluster Headache | 145
    Paroxysmal Hemicrania | 150
    Short-Lasting Unilateral Neuralgiform Headache | 151
    Hemicrania Continua | 152

New Daily Persistent Headache | 153

Treating Unusual Headaches: A Success and a Failure | 154

15. Head Injuries and Headache | 157

Concussion | 157

The Post-concussive Syndrome | 159

16. How to Communicate with Your Medical Team | 163

The Initial Visit | 164

What to Do Between Visits | 166

The Follow-Up Visit | 167

If You Have Problems with the Medical Team | 170

17. Migraine Resources | 171

ACKNOWLEDGMENTS | 175
ABOUT THE AUTHORS | 177
INDEX | 181

PREFACE: WHY WE WROTE THIS BOOK

Around half to three-quarters of all adults in the world have had a significant headache in the last year. And as much as 4% of the world's population has a headache on 15 or more days every month. This amounts to more than 200 million people who have headache on more days than not!

Headache conditions affect people of all ages, races, income levels, and geographical areas. The World Health Organization has found that migraine, the major cause of recurring headaches, is one of the world's leading causes of disability, not to mention suffering.

If you are reading this book you either suffer from headaches or care about someone who has troubling headaches. People who struggle with headaches often look "fine" and receive little sympathy. People with serious headache problems often wait for months to see specialists in the field, if they are even referred to such specialists by their primary physicians. Even after their evaluation by a specialist, headache sufferers often remain uncertain about their diagnosis, why they have their headaches, and which of the many treatment options might be best for them. This book will address those concerns in a common-sense and straightforward yet comprehensive fashion.

Our book begins by addressing a question most headache sufferers have: "Is this migraine, or is it a more dangerous type of headache?" This worry is sometimes such a concern that people with headache are actually afraid to seek help. However, as a survey of patients' concerns has shown, it is the most important question most patients want answered.

After tackling that concern, we discuss the nature and causes of migraines, the impact they have on sufferers' lives, the best ways to "escape" from a migraine attack, and the best ways to prevent migraines from occurring. We delve into the many medical approaches to migraine but also pay heed to something many of our patients are passionate about: how to control their headaches without medication.

Following this, we discuss headaches in children and adolescents, the special circumstances facing pregnant and breastfeeding women with migraine, and the difficulties posed by chronic migraine—that is, migraine occurring on 15 or more days a month. We also devote space to other important questions that arise in managing your headaches: how to measure success and how to make decisions about new and experimental treatments. After discussing the most common type of headache, we then cover some unusual causes of headache and consider headaches and other problems that arise after head injuries. Having the right caregivers is important, and in our last two chapters we address how to communicate with your medical team and tell you about resources that will help you gather information about your care on your own.

Both of us have been evaluating and managing people with headaches for more than 30 years. We have observed virtually every type of headache imaginable and have explored countless treatment ideas. We have learned that every patient is unique but that there are certain predictably effective approaches to caring for the various headache types. In writing this book we have tried to share as much as we can of what we have learned with you. Unfortunately there is still much to learn about headache disorders and there are gaps in our ability to manage some aspects of headache problems. There is nonetheless hope, as research centers are making real progress in headache medicine.

The most important thing we want to stress is that you should not give up hope that there is a way for your headaches to improve. We have found that with proper care, it is the rare patient indeed who will not see enough improvement to regain at least a good measure of control and autonomy.

Mo Levin and Tom Ward

UNDERSTANDING YOUR MIGRAINES

Chapter 1

What Type of Headache Do I Have?

Whether you have had headaches for a long time or just recently began to be bothered by them, you probably wonder what type of headache condition you have. (That is probably why you are reading this book). Even people who have been definitively diagnosed with a particular headache type often wonder if there is something potentially dangerous happening, especially if their pain is not responding to treatment. In fact, headaches *can* be a clue to an underlying medical problem in the head or neck or even elsewhere in the body. Competent doctors and other healthcare providers know this and are generally very careful to think about all of the possible causes when their patients bring up their headaches.

There are many different kinds of headaches and many causes of pain around the head, neck, and face. The International Headache Society has created a system for classifying headache conditions that includes over 200 headache types, called the International Classification of Headache Disorders. This classification system helps doctors diagnose headaches based on the signs and symptoms patients are experiencing. Careful evaluation of patients with headaches is important so that the most serious causes can be quickly ruled out. You may first visit your general physician or even a doctor in the emergency room, but it is sometimes best to seek out a headache specialist for the most effective diagnosis and treatment (especially if your headaches are causing you to miss work, family, social, and leisure activities or are diminishing your ability to participate in these activities).

Headaches are generally divided into two broad categories: primary headaches and secondary headaches. **Primary headaches** are those that have their origin in some altered but not life-threatening activity in the brain. These include *migraine* (by far the most common primary headache type that comes to medical attention), *tension-type headache* (the most common headache type), *cluster headache*, and a number of much less common varieties of recurring, non-life-threatening headaches. **Secondary headaches** are those considered to be due to medical problems in the head, neck, or elsewhere that cause head pain for one reason or another. Some of these causes, such as infections, tumors, and body chemistry changes, can have serious consequences and must be addressed quickly. Other causes of secondary headaches, such as previous head trauma or arthritis, tend to be chronic and, while not life-threatening, nonetheless cause disability.

In this chapter we will take a journey through the world of headache-causing conditions to help you sort through the possibilities, some of which you might have considered. That is not to say we can enable you to diagnose your headaches with certainty—that will occur when you see a well-trained clinician, who will listen to your history, examine you, and perhaps arrange diagnostic testing such as blood tests or imaging of the brain and head with magnetic resonance imaging (MRI) or computerized tomography (CT) (Fig. 1.1). We hope this section of the book will give you a bit of a head start (sorry for the pun) in understanding your headaches.

Primary Headaches

Migraine

There are several categories of primary headaches (see Box 1.1), but the most important is **migraine**. Chapter 2 will flesh out the

(a)

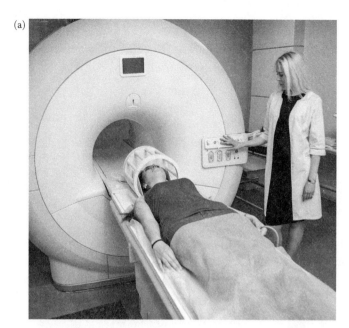

(b)

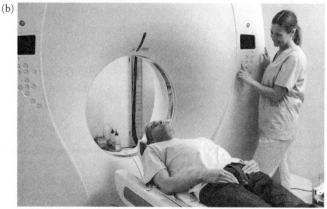

FIG. 1.1 (a) A patient undergoing magnetic resonance imaging (MRI). People who are uncomfortable in closed spaces may find this procedure a little disturbing, but their discomfort is easily treated with mild sedatives like lorazepam. (b) A patient having a computerized tomography (CT) scan. CT is less constricting and faster than MRI, but generally less useful in diagnosing headaches. (Images courtesy of shutterstock.com.)

> **BOX 1.1 Primary Headaches (Not Due to Something Else)**
>
> • Migraine
> • Tension-type headache
> • Cluster headache (and other trigeminal autonomic cephalalgias)
> • Other headaches, including exertion-related headaches

features of these very common headaches: how they occur, what they feel like, and how you know if you are a migraine sufferer, also known as a *migraineur*. But a simple definition of migraine would be something like *recurring severe headaches lasting at least a few hours, generally accompanied by nausea, sensitivity to light and sound, or both*. Migraines tend to run in families, tend to affect women more than men, and generally start in a person's teens or twenties. The severity of migraine pain can range from mild to very severe, but usually migraines are bad enough to lead people to at least sometimes miss work or school and to feel the need to do something to relieve the pain.

Tension-Type Headaches

Tension-type headaches, on the other hand, tend to be milder, although they too can be intrusive enough to make a pretty big impact on a person's day. They are often described as "all over the head" or as a "band of pain around the head." Fortunately, they generally respond to over-the-counter pills like acetaminophen (Tylenol) or ibuprofen (Advil, Motrin). They tend not to involve the migraine symptoms of nausea or sensitivity to light and sound. Tension-type headaches affect men as often as women and may start a bit later in life than migraines.

An odd thing about migraine and tension-type headaches is that some people seem to get both of these types of headaches, although at different times. Let's take a look at a real patient with recurring bothersome headaches (as with all the patients discussed in this book, we do not use her real name):

Ann is a 34-year-old mother of two elementary school–age children who works part-time as an office manager. She tells her primary care physician about her increasingly frequent headaches. They seem to take two forms: One is a very severe throbbing headache, usually around her temple and eye on one or the other side, which makes her feel nauseated. She cannot go to work or do much of anything when she has this kind of headache, and she generally has to go lie down in a dark, quiet room. She is guaranteed to have one of these headaches around the time of her menstrual periods, but they occur at other times too. Aspirin, acetaminophen, and ibuprofen don't seem to help much, and she just has to tough the headache out until she goes to sleep in the evening. Ann has the second kind of headache a little more frequently, but these headaches are milder (though still aggravating—she says they are "nagging") and seem to go away eventually with ibuprofen or massage. They occur when she has not slept enough or is under more stress than usual. Taking the two types together, it seems to Ann that she is having some kind of headache several days each week, although she cannot give an exact frequency.

Did you recognize the more severe headaches as migraines and the milder, less severe ones as tension-type headaches? Both are bothersome to Ann, but the migraines are absolutely disabling. Does she have two independent medical conditions? Are the two headache types linked in some way? These questions are actually hotly debated by headache researchers. The important point is that *both* headache types need to be addressed in this patient, as both are clearly detracting in significant ways from her quality of life.

Cluster Headaches

On the extreme end of the headache pain spectrum are **cluster headaches**, considered by most headache specialists to be the worst headache anyone can experience. This headache type is fairly rare, although every neurologist has seen a number of patients with cluster headaches sometime during his or her career. The pain, generally located in the area around one eye, is excruciating, but thankfully attacks last only around an hour or so. The typical cluster headache is accompanied by tearing from the eye on the side of the headache, nasal congestion or drainage, and the urge to pace back and forth. Cluster headaches are more common in men and tend to arise at a later age than migraine. The term "cluster" arose because patients with this type of headache usually have long headache-free intervals (typically months) punctuated by several weeks of one or more headaches per day. These clusters of days with severe bouts of pain can be highly demoralizing to sufferers and have even been known to trigger thoughts of suicide.

One of the strangest things about cluster headaches is their excellent response to breathing pure oxygen for several minutes. Also, fortunately there are some very effective preventive treatments for these devastating headaches, including prednisone (a steroid medication), verapamil (a medication used for high blood pressure), and lithium, a medication used for psychiatric diseases. (It is not unusual to use "non-headache drugs" to treat headaches—headache specialists use many medications initially developed for other illnesses very effectively.) There is usually a dramatic response to injections of the headache drug sumatriptan (Imitrex), with the pain disappearing completely within a few minutes.

Cluster headaches occupy a category in the headache disorders classification called "trigeminal autonomic cephalalgias." This category includes several types of headache that resemble cluster headache but tend to be briefer (lasting minutes or even just seconds). There is another headache type in this category— *hemicrania continua*—that, like cluster headache, affects only one side of the head, but which is incessant unless the patient is treated with a very specific antidote, the anti-inflammatory medication called indomethacin. We will consider the trigeminal autonomic cephalalgias in more detail in Chapter 14.

Rare Primary Headache Conditions

There are also a number of other rare headache conditions, like **cough headaches**; **hypnic headaches** (also known as "alarm clock headaches," because they occur in the middle of the night); **exertional headaches,** which occur only with exercise; **nummular headaches** (named because of the small, coin-sized area of pain in the scalp—the term derives from *nummus,* which is the Latin word for "coin"); and **headaches related to sexual activity**. Fortunately, most of these conditions are treatable.

Let's have a look at a particularly frustrating case in this category:

Sam is a 40-year-old contractor who reluctantly tells his physician about some very upsetting headaches he has been having recently. During sex, he can experience severe "crushing" headaches that seem to come from the "center of my head" and feel like "something is going to explode." When these headaches occur, they seem to happen close to or at the time of orgasm. He has to stop and hold his head in his hands for several minutes until the pain lessens. Gradually, the pain dissipates, after which he just feels "drained." The headaches do not always happen when he and his wife have sex, but the fear of them has significantly cut into their sex life. They have experimented with different positions, hoping that they will find a way to prevent the headaches, but this has not worked. He is worried about what these headaches are due to but is more concerned about the impact on his marriage.

This of course is the headache related to sexual activity, a rather mysterious condition that for obvious reasons is highly upsetting and downright scary. The first occurrence of such a headache should be viewed as a true emergency, because the pain resembles what people can experience with bleeding in the brain and other life-threatening neurological illnesses. With a recurring pattern like Sam had, concern for danger is minimal, and fortunately there are some effective treatments.

Secondary Headaches

As we said, there are many causes of headaches, some of which must be recognized rapidly to ensure that you get the right treatment in a timely way. Box 1.2 lists the major categories that physicians think about when considering possible causes of headaches. However—and this is important to remember— the vast majority of people with headaches have a non-life-threatening (although of course still bothersome) condition like migraine or tension-type headache. Your physician will listen to your description of your headaches and examine you to find

---

**BOX 1.2 Secondary Headaches (Caused by
Another Disorder)**

- Post-traumatic headaches
- Headaches due to stroke and other blood vessel diseases
- Headaches related to abnormal intracranial pressure or masses
- Headaches due to use of drugs or other substances or to withdrawal from same
- Headaches due to brain and other infections
- Headaches due to high blood pressure, thyroid problems, and other metabolic conditions
- Headaches due to neck disorders
- Headaches due to disorders of eyes, ears, nose and sinuses, teeth, and jaw
- Headaches due to psychiatric causes

---

clues that one of these secondary headaches may be occurring. (Box 1.3 lists typical clues we look for.) Let's review the major categories of secondary headaches.

Post-traumatic Headaches

Injuries to the head can lead to a number of long-term problems. We are learning more and more about the consequences of head trauma from injured athletes and injured soldiers returning from war zones who describe symptoms ranging from memory and concentration problems to sleep and emotional difficulties to a number of pain complaints. The most common and persistent symptom after a mild-to-moderate head injury is headache,

> **BOX 1.3** Features That Suggest Searching for an
> Underlying Medical Cause of Headaches
>
> A new headache type or a clear change in the pattern of
> headaches
> Fever
> Change in sensation
> Change in strength
> Gait problems
> Confusion or memory loss
> Headache worsens with position changes
> Headache is always in the same place
> Chronic illness such as AIDS or cancer
> Onset of headaches in middle age or later
> Pregnancy
> Taking anticoagulant medication

which can take a number of forms, including migraine-like head-aches with throbbing pain and nausea. In a number of patients with **post-traumatic headaches**, previously existing headaches like migraine are seemingly made worse by head injury. Sadly, the headaches these individuals experience are only a small part of their post-traumatic problems. You will read more about this growing problem in Chapter 15.

Blood Vessels and Headaches

Stroke, generally resulting from blockage of one or more brain arteries, leads to headache about a third of the time, but a number of other problems with brain arteries (and sometimes veins) can also produce headaches. One well-known, and scary, possibility is an aneurysm (a tiny pouch) on an artery that is either swelling or bleeding. ***Subarachnoid hemorrhage*** (bleeding from an aneurysm) generally causes sudden, very severe headache, bad enough to lead people to call 911 and get to an ER quickly. If this rare but serious condition does not receive medical attention it can lead to sudden death. Another cause of headache due to abnormal blood vessels in the brain is ***vasculitis***, an inflammation of brain arteries that can mimic other headache types, even migraine. This condition is diagnosed with CT or MRI of the brain arteries, blood testing, and evaluation of spinal fluid. One more blood vessel–related condition that can cause headaches is an ***arteriovenous malformation (AVM)*** in the brain or tissues surrounding the brain. An AVM is a relatively unusual abnormality consisting of a tangled mass of arteries and veins thought in most cases to be present from birth (Fig. 1.2).

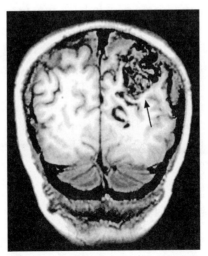

FIG. 1.2 Brain MRI image of an arteriovenous malformation (AVM), indicated by the arrow, that led to headaches and seizures. (From Rustam Al-Shahi, Charles Warlow. A systematic review of the frequency and prognosis of arteriovenous malformations of the brain in adults. *Brain*. Oxford University Press. Pg. 124. 2001-10-01. By permission of Oxford University Press.)

Intracranial Hypertension Headaches

An odd headache type sometimes called **benign intracranial hypertension** is due to abnormally high pressure in the head. Pain occurs because certain very sensitive membranes around the brain are stretched as a result of the high pressure. This condition isn't really "benign," as it can cause loss of vision in addition to some very severe headaches. The only way to diagnose it is by doing a lumbar puncture (spinal tap) to measure the pressure of the spinal fluid. This headache used to be known as *pseudotumor cerebri*, because the pain and other symptoms that patients experienced resembled those in patients with brain tumors.

Low Intracranial Pressure Headaches

On the other hand, some people have **low intracranial pressure,** which can also lead to head pain by distorting or stretching the highly sensitive linings around the brain, due to "sagging" of the entire brain downward: the brain, which normally floats in the spinal fluid, instead sags. These people tend to get an increase in head pain when they stand up and nearly total relief of their headache when they lie down. This condition is also diagnosed with a lumbar puncture, but strong clues can sometimes be seen on an MRI scan of the brain.

Brain Malformations

Malformations of the skull and brain can also cause headache. One in particular, the **Chiari malformation**, is not that rare and can easily be seen on MRI scans of the head. One clue to the presence of this malformation is headache and neck pain induced by coughing or straining.

Brain Tumors

Brain tumors, whether benign or malignant, may cause headache as an initial sign of trouble. Many patients with new headache worry about this possibility, but probability is in their favor—only a small minority of headaches are ultimately found to be due to tumors or other masses in the brain. At any rate, MRI scanning of the head—a painless and essentially risk-free procedure—quickly rules out such possibilities. Your doctor will know to look for warning signs like weakness or loss of sensation in part of your body, vision changes, trouble communicating, or significant difficulty with cognitive tasks. Without any such clues, it is highly unlikely your headaches are due to any of these serious causes.

Seizures and Headaches

Epileptic seizures often induce headaches, but not as a person's only symptom. If there is any suspicion of seizures, a neurologist can generally rule them out pretty quickly by hearing your description of headache spells and, if necessary, ordering an electroencephalogram (EEG) (Fig. 1.3). An EEG, like MRI and CT scanning, is a painless, essentially risk-free procedure; electrical sensors are attached to your scalp and connected to a device that records brain activity over about 30 minutes.

Medication Overuse Headaches

Many medications can cause headaches—but you already know this, because it seems that the side effect listing for just about any medication includes headache. In reality, few medications cause significant headache in people who otherwise have no

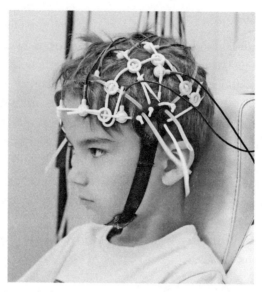

FIG. 1.3 A patient having an electroencephalogram (EEG). This test is painless but does take about an hour and is most revealing if the subject is able to fall asleep during it. Because of this we usually ask patients to stay up late the evening before the test and wake up early on the day of the test. (Image courtesy of shutterstock.com.)

tendency toward migraine or other headache. A bigger problem, though, is the so-called ***medication overuse headache*** (formerly known as *analgesic rebound headache*), which occurs when people with migraine consume painkiller medication more frequently than the recommended 2 or 3 days per week. The way this happens is not entirely understood, but it can be a very frustrating problem for both patients and their medical teams, since treating headaches can actually make them worse when you don't stick to careful guidelines.

Here is a real story of how medication overuse can arise and quickly spin out of control:

Amy is a 38-year-old new-car salesperson. She is a high producer at her dealership and has been very successful financially. What her manager and associates do not know is that she is experiencing headaches nearly every day and has to resort to a number of medications during the day to maintain her fast-paced routine. She began having headaches in her teens, usually around the time of her menstrual periods. They have always involved some degree of nausea. They were infrequent for a few years, but in her twenties they began to occur more frequently. Excedrin used to be very effective for treating her headaches, but now she has to use four tablets at a time to just "take the edge off." Aspirin and ibuprofen were of some help in the past but no longer are. Amy says that a medication called Fioricet was "my lifesaver" when her physician prescribed it several years ago. It reduced the pain significantly, but over the past year, she convinced her physician to prescribe the form that also contains codeine in higher and higher quantities, and she admits that she now needs about 80 tablets per month to keep headache pain at bay. Her doctor refuses to increase these amounts, even though at current levels she runs out of pills toward the end of each month. She has used some of her husband's Percocet and thinks it is an effective medication for her, but it too is seemingly less potent than it was at first. She wakes up every morning with a headache and has to take the Fioricet quickly to keep it from escalating. Over the last several months, Amy has had to go to the ER a few times for particularly severe headaches. She became tearful when relating that one of the ER doctors seemed to treat her like a "drug addict": "They don't realize that I am just taking the pills so I can function!"

This is almost certainly a serious case of medication overuse headaches. Not only has Amy developed tolerance to (reduced effectiveness of) the headache-relieving medications, but they are actually causing some if not all of her headaches. It is a classic vicious cycle. Clues for the insightful physician are (1) the increased need for the medications, (2) the increasing frequency of headaches, and (3) the presence of headache every morning (when the pain medication has left the system). Most patients realize there is a problem when they notice the large collection of pill bottles they carry around and the constant need to refill their prescriptions. The only way to help patients like Amy is to actually "retrain" their brains to accept less and less medication and to find a way to prevent headaches with non-medicinal and carefully limited medicinal strategies, which we will discuss in later chapters.

Recreational Drug Use and Headaches

Along entirely different lines, a growing cause of headaches is the array of mind-altering drugs available (some legal), like "bath salts" and "smoked incense," that can directly cause head pain. Some, like marijuana, have even been promoted as remedies for migraine and other headaches, though without any proof yet. Psychedelics like psilocybin mushrooms and LSD may cause headaches in some people as well, although there is some evidence that they may actually help some people who experience cluster headaches. (We believe it is best to wait for further evidence and legalization before using these options, however.) Opioid drugs like street heroin and prescription painkiller pills like OxyContin and Vicodin have pain-reducing properties but are all very likely to eventually cause headache, either due to withdrawal or via the mechanism of medication overuse headache.

Medical Illness and Headaches

Infection in the brain (**encephalitis**) or in the linings around the brain (**meningitis**) often causes significant head pain. In these cases the patient has usually had good health, with no headache problems, until recently experiencing changes in behavior, new headaches, or both. Other infections, like sinus infections or even pneumonia or the flu, can cause headaches along with their other symptoms. All of these potential causes must be considered when evaluating headache, since it is crucial to discover any infectious disease that can be treated with antibiotics. General **metabolic problems** can sometimes cause headaches, the most familiar examples being thyroid abnormalities and poorly controlled diabetes. High blood pressure can sometimes lead to headaches, but probably not as often as commonly believed. Other **head and facial problems** can lead to headache, such as eye disease, dental disease, and jaw problems (like temporomandibular joint disorder, or TMD). **Neck problems** are also a source of headache and in fact explain a number of headaches in elderly people with severe arthritic conditions of the neck. This form of headache is referred to as **cervicogenic headache.**

Mental Illness and Headaches

It has long been observed that people with headaches are likely to suffer from anxiety disorders, depression, or both. Because of this, it has often been postulated that some headaches are due to forms of mental illness. This has never really been shown to be true, although many people, including many physicians, mistakenly consider psychiatric and psychological causes of headaches to be common. On the other hand, depression and other mental illnesses can probably *worsen* headaches like migraine and tension-type headache. And clearly, headaches may worsen underlying mental illness, since they can make life so difficult for the sufferer.

Neuralgia

Finally, there is a category of pain called **neuralgia,** which results from a malfunction in a nerve (or group of nerves) that signals pain to the brain even when there is no apparent reason for pain. This situation, also known as "false message pain," results from nerve damage or irritation. Head pain can arise when the nerve in question is in the face, head, or upper neck. The nerve irritation can be due to a viral infection, compression by a local blood vessel, or trauma to the nerve. Whatever the cause, the pain can become excruciating. The head and facial pain caused by neuralgia is usually severe but very brief (although it can occur many times per day), with a "stabbing" or "electrical" quality, and tends to respond to medical treatment quite well. A well-known type of neuralgia is **trigeminal neuralgia** (named after the trigeminal nerve, the major nerve of the face), which causes one-sided facial pain.

Summary

There are many causes of headache. Most headache patients seeking medical advice have migraine, which you will read more about in later chapters, but certain types of secondary headaches, like those due to head trauma and those due to medications or other substances, can masquerade as primary headaches and must be identified correctly to ensure the best results from treatment. Fortunately, most secondary headache conditions are easy for physicians to diagnose and treat, particularly if they have some experience in the field and are comfortable with the diagnostic tests we have discussed above.

Chapter 2

Do I Have Migraine?

Let's look at four clinical stories first, to give us some examples with which to consider the important question "Do I have migraine?"

> Rebecca is a 47-year-old registered nurse who has had "sinus headaches" since about the age of 14. She describes them as a sensation of fullness in her face with some mild accompanying nausea. They are infrequent (only 2–3 attacks monthly), and in the past her family physician has treated them with antibiotics. They usually get better in 2–3 days. Sinus surgery has not improved matters. During a recent attack an otolaryngologist (an eye, nears, and throat physician) obtained a CT scan of her sinuses, and it was absolutely normal with no sign of infection. Rebecca was then referred to the headache clinic. Further inquiry revealed that her mother had a history of similar "sinus headaches." Rebecca's 13-year-old daughter, Beth, who just started having periods this year, has begun having occasional headaches related to her menses.

What is going on with Beth?

> Beth was a "colicky" baby. As a child she suffered from motion sickness, and she has fainted twice (once in the church choir, and once while having her blood drawn for

laboratory tests). She has found that the day before her period starts she will sometimes wake up with a moderately severe headache that can last 2–3 days. Tylenol sometimes controls the headaches, but other times they can become severe; she has had to come home from school twice because of the headaches. She prefers to lie down in a dark, quiet room when headache occurs. The headache is over her forehead and sinuses, so she wonders if she too has sinus headaches, like her mother.

Our third patient's headache pattern shows some features not seen in Rebecca or Beth:

Alexander is a 30-year-old bank loan officer. As a child, he did not suffer from significant headaches, but for the past several years he has been troubled by 3–4 severe headaches per month. A day or so before each attack he finds himself yawning a lot and is irritable. He recognizes that this is how he feels shortly before the onset of his headaches. Sometimes he craves chocolate before the attacks, and he wonders if stress or a lack of sleep may trigger some of the headaches. Before some of the more severe episodes he may see flashing silvery lights or zigzag lines for several minutes. His headaches are usually on the right side of his head, but very occasionally they can be on the left side. During the headaches he becomes nauseated, and on one occasion only he has vomited. The overhead lights at the bank are bothersome to him even if he does not have a headache.

Our fourth patient has a history of what she believes to be migraine, but her pattern has changed over time:

Mary has been troubled by headaches since college. She is now 52 years old. Initially they occurred twice a month but could last up to 3 days. She never found over-the-counter medications particularly helpful in controlling the headache, but she has used narcotics for the more severe attacks and they seem to dull the headaches. She has increased her use of narcotics over the years and now finds the headaches are occurring more than 25 days each month. In fact, it is rare for her to have a truly headache-free day. Her severe headaches involve the entire head and are "pounding." She is nauseated during the severe attacks but wonders if that is a result of the medication. When she is not having a "migraine" she usually has a milder headache, mainly in the back of her head, that she experiences as a mild "pressure." Her doctor has recently diagnosed her with depression and recommended an antidepressant medication.

We know we said four cases. But here is a fifth case, with some similarities to the previous ones. Do you notice one significant different feature?

Mark is a 63-year-old man with no prior history of headaches. About 2 weeks after having the "flu" he developed a headache, which has persisted for 7 months. The headache just began one day and has never gone away. The pain is constant but varies in severity from mild to severe. It is in his entire head, and when it is severe his head pounds and he is nauseated. Sometimes he finds lights and sound unpleasant; he then lies down in a dark, quiet room. His family physician has not been able to find any medication that helps, nor has a specialist in "headache medicine." Extensive testing has yielded only normal results.

At the end of the chapter, we will apply what we have learned to see which of these five patients are suffering from migraine.

What Is Migraine?

The majority of patients who come to see a doctor with inter-
mittent, occasionally disabling headaches will turn out to have
migraine. According to the World Health Organization migraine
is the third most common of all diseases and the eighth most disabling overall (fourth for women). To deal with this condition,
the first order of business is to make a correct diagnosis. The
International Classification of Headache Disorders (ICHD) is the
standard by which headache disorders are designated. Here is what
the third, most recent edition of the ICHD says about migraine:

Description: Recurrent headache disorder manifesting in
attacks lasting 4–72 hours. Typical characteristics of the
headaches are unilateral location, pulsating quality, moderate or severe intensity, aggravation by routine physical
activity and association with nausea and/or extreme sensitivity to light or sound (photophobia and phonophobia).
Diagnostic criteria:
A. At least five attacks fulfilling criteria B–D
B. Headache attacks lasting 4–72 hours (untreated or
unsuccessfully treated)
C. Headache has at least two of the following four
characteristics:
1. unilateral location
2. pulsating quality
3. moderate or severe pain intensity
4. aggravation by or causing avoidance of routine
physical activity (e.g., walking or climbing stairs)
D. During headache at least one of the following:
1. nausea and/or vomiting
2. photophobia and phonophobia
E. Not better accounted for by another ICHD-3 diagnosis.

Migraine often begins in childhood or the teenage years. It is uncommon for it to begin after the age of 40 years. In children the attacks are often briefer and more easily relieved by sleep. It is about equally common in boys and girls, but after puberty it becomes about twice as frequent in females, and by about the age of 35 it is three times as common in women as men (present in about 18% vs. 6% of the respective populations). After menopause the attacks lessen in frequency and severity, and by the age of 70 the pain usually stops. Fig. 2.1 shows the prevalence of migraine throughout the life cycle.

Not all headaches are migraines, and there are a number of conditions—some serious—that mimic migraines. Mass lesions such as brain tumors certainly can cause headaches, as can other conditions we reviewed in the last chapter. So it is very important to make sure something else is not the cause of your

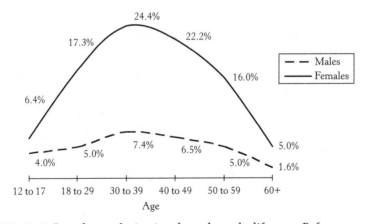

FIG. 2.1 Prevalence of migraine throughout the life span. Before puberty, the differences between boys' and girls' rates of migraine are negligible. This begins to change dramatically after puberty; during midlife, around three times as many women as men suffer from migraine. (From *Wolff's Headache and Other Pain*, 8th edition, edited by Stephen Silberstein, Richard Lipton, and David Dodick [2008]: Fig. 4.2. By permission of Oxford University Press.)

BOX 2.1 Conditions That Mimic Migraine

New daily persistent headache: headache that begins one day and lasts at least 3 months

Post-traumatic headache: headache that begins or, if pre-existing, worsens following head trauma; may look like any other type of headache, including migraine

Hemicrania continua: a constant one-sided headache that varies in severity; may look like attacks of migraine when it worsens

Mass lesions: infrequent migraine mimic due to an abnormal structure in the brain such as a tumor or an arteriovenous malformation (AVM), a collection of abnormal blood vessels

---

headaches. While it is reassuring if the headaches occur intermittently and you are absolutely fine in between the attacks, doctors should be particularly concerned about patients with headaches that begin after the age of 40 or before the age of 5, who have abnormalities on their neurological examinations, or who have headaches that are *always* on the same side. Headaches that are constant or are worsening are cause for concern as well. Box 2.1 lists several important mimics of migraine.

Migraine Triggers

Migraine is notorious for having triggers. As a rule of thumb, a trigger is something that, when the migraine sufferer is exposed to it, is followed by a migraine attack more often than not (usually within a few minutes to hours). So sometimes one might have exposure to a trigger and not get an attack. While some patients do not have obvious triggers, most patients feel they do.

Avoiding triggers has been advocated since the time of Hippocrates. However, doing this is not as simple as it sounds. Food cravings and other feelings that occur during the prodrome (pre-headache phase, also called the warning or premonitory phase) of a migraine attack (see Fig. 2.2) can lead to confusion about what is and is not a trigger. For example, we know many patients who begin to feel the need to have something sweet prior to the onset of their migraines. They grab something like a chocolate bar, and later the headache begins. They might draw the conclusion that the chocolate caused the migraine, but in fact the craving was merely part of the onset of the migraine. For those patients who experience the prodrome of a migraine, it occurs days to hours before an attack and may consist of food cravings, neck pain, irritability, fatigue, yawning, or euphoria or energy. Some patients eventually recognize these symptoms as signs of an impending attack. For those patients, these symptoms represent an opportunity to prepare for or perhaps even prevent an attack.

Patients will sometimes find published lists of migraine triggers and avoid them, even if they are not their own triggers. We have listed some of the more common triggers in Box 2.2. One

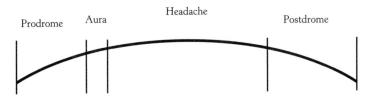

FIG. 2.2 Phases of a migraine attack: prodrome, aura (if present), headache, and postdrome.

BOX 2.2 Some Migraine Triggers

Weather (particularly, rapid changes in atmospheric pressure)

Travel (at high altitude or across time zones)

Menstrual periods or hormonal changes

Stress and anxiety

Physical exertion

Sleep deprivation or changes

Head trauma

Odors (perfumes, fumes from fuel or solvents)

Dietary factors: delaying or skipping a meal, fasting, dehydration; for some patients, certain aged cheeses (depending on amount of the chemical tyramine), alcohol, monosodium glutamate (goes by many other names), cold foods (may cause "ice cream headache"), certain aged or processed meats (may have high levels of tyramine, nitrates, or both), caffeine

---

very important trigger for many patients is delaying a meal. We should emphasize that food triggers of migraine are not due to food *allergy*, so testing for food allergy is not helpful. Other triggers include certain medications, menstrual periods (and for some women, ovulation, which occurs about 2 weeks before menses, when there is also a drop in blood estrogen levels), certain odors, glare, alcohol, gluten (in individuals who have gluten intolerance), loud noise, sleep disturbances, traveling at altitude or rapid descent from altitude, weather changes, and stress. In fact, stress is usually number one on patients' lists of triggers, but of course "stress" means different things to each of us.

Remember: not all triggers are equally potent. In some circumstances a single trigger might not be sufficient to result in a migraine, but multiple triggers occurring together might be almost guaranteed to provoke a migraine attack.

Migraine Aura

About a quarter of migraine sufferers also experience an "aura." Although often thought of as occurring before migraine headaches, auras can occur without an associated headache or occur before, during, or even after any type of headache. Most often, aura is a visual phenomenon that lasts for 5–60 minutes before a migraine attack. The aura may consist of an enlarging blind spot (hole in your vision), perhaps with a shimmering edge; flashing lights; zigzag lines; stars; "heat waves"; or other things. Less often, an aura may be tingling that typically starts in the hand and gradually, over minutes, ascends the arm, moves to the face, and even goes inside the mouth, where it may make your tongue go numb. Even less common are weakness on one side of the body, speech disturbances, and confusion. Other symptoms can include vertigo, double vision, clumsiness or staggering, sleepiness, and tingling on both sides of the body. On first occurrence these symptoms can be quite frightening, but over time the migraineur often comes to realize that their appearance may herald an imminent severe headache and represent an opportunity to start treatment.

Migraine Features

The pain of migraine may begin on just one side of the head (the classic presentation) or both sides. It can vary from mild to severe and may be experienced as pounding, pressure, or sharp pain. Many people also develop nausea, vomiting, or both and sensitivity to light, sound, and even smells. To deal with their symptoms, patients tend to lie down in a dark, quiet room and, if unable to stop their headache attack, will try to sleep. In adults unsuccessfully treated migraine attacks typically last 4–72 hours; attacks in children tend to be briefer. Episodes lasting longer than 72 hours are called *status migrainosus*. During these prolonged attacks the migraineur may become dehydrated, especially if he or she has been vomiting, and sleep-deprived.

The Aftermath of a Migraine Attack

Once the pain phase of a migraine resolves, you may experience the "postdrome." You may feel sore all over, fatigued, dehydrated, sleep-deprived, or just really "wiped out." There is gradual improvement until the next attack. Depending on the duration and severity of the pain phase, the postdrome can last from a few hours to several days. After that, you tend to go back to your usual state but may have mild lingering symptoms.

Medical Conditions Associated with Migraine

Migraine sufferers tend to have certain other conditions more often than people who do not have migraines. Individuals who eventually develop migraines may be more likely to have colic as infants and to experience "cyclic vomiting," "abdominal migraine," and some types of vertigo as children. In fact symptoms of vertigo and imbalance are not at all uncommon in migraine patients and sometimes cause serious problems. Migraineurs often have motion sickness and a tendency to faint and may have cold hands and cold feet (Raynaud's phenomenon). Depression and anxiety as well as other psychiatric conditions are more common in migraine patients. Migraineurs are often poor sleepers, which can seem normal to them until they acquire bed partners who sleep better than they do. Migraine also has weak associations with seizures (epilepsy) and stroke. Asthma is also more common in people with migraine.

Migraine can be classified by how often it occurs: migraine fewer than 15 days per month is called "episodic" and migraine 15 or more days per month "chronic." Certain treatments may work better for one of these groups than the other. Chronic migraine can sometimes be associated with other conditions, such as thyroid disorders, too much caffeine intake, psychiatric problems, head trauma, sleep disturbance, or medication overuse (analgesic rebound). Box 2.3 lists some conditions associated with higher migraine frequency.

Migraine is generally inherited. Sometimes the family history suggests otherwise, but studies suggest that histories

---

BOX 2.3 Conditions That Worsen (Increase Frequency of) Migraine

Obesity (the more overweight, the greater the effect)
Snoring or sleep apnea
Psychological issues or stressful life events (moving; issues at work, with children, or in one's marriage)
Head injury
Thyroid disease (high or low thyroid function)

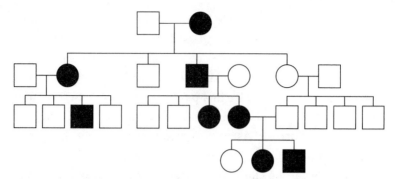

FIG. 2.3 A genogram (or pedigree) of a family with migraine. Circles indicate females, and squares males. A circle and square attached with a horizontal line indicate mates who produced children, who appear below them. A solid (black) circle or square signifies that the person has or had migraine.

known to the patient are often wrong. Sometimes migraineurs outgrow the tendency as they age and do not mention it to younger family members. Also, migraine is sometimes misdiagnosed as "sinus headache" or other types of headaches (e.g., due to "eye strain" or temporomandibular joint [TMJ] disorders). While keeping these considerations in mind, a good way to investigate this issue is to create a "genogram" (much like a family tree) showing your family history for migraines (Fig. 2.3).

Given the fairly high frequency of head injury in modern society, it is notable that such injury can cause headaches that resemble migraine. Headache is a prominent feature of "postconcussive syndrome" and also occurs following whiplash events.

Diagnosing Migraine: Our Examples

Let's go back to our five headache cases from the start of the chapter and see who had migraine.

Rebecca, the first patient, had migraine but it was previously misdiagnosed as "sinus headache." Her daughter, Beth, was a "colicky" baby (which we have noted can be associated with migraine) and inherited her mother's migraineur tendency. Rebecca and Beth both respond well to treatment with sumatriptan (Imitrex), which is a well-known migraine treatment (one of the so-called triptans).

Alexander, the third patient, also had migraine, with a prodrome that he recognized and, with some of the headaches, an aura as well. The chocolate cravings were actually part of his prodrome and not a trigger: he got migraines whether or not he ate the chocolate he desired.

Mary, our fourth patient, also had migraine, which initially was episodic (occurring less than half the month) but had become chronic. Sadly, she was taking more pills but having more headaches. She likely had medication overuse headache, which occurs in migraineurs who use too much symptomatic medication (in her case narcotics). Usually, as the amount of medication used increases, the headaches become more frequent and often

---

BOX 2.4 Self-Assessment Checklist for Diagnosing Migraine (Not All Features Are Necessary)

☐ Attacks of headache lasting 4–72 hours (briefer in children)
☐ Disability during attacks, returning to normal until next attack
☐ Nausea during some of the attacks
☐ Sensitivity to light, sound, or both
☐ Other family members with migraine

harder to control (see Chapter 1). Stopping the problematic medication resulted in great improvement in her headache situation.

Lastly, Mark did not have migraine. While he came to our clinic with that diagnosis, he instead had "new daily persistent headache." This type of headache just begins one day, sometimes after a viral infection or surgery, and may have features of migraine, tension-type headache, or both. It usually does not respond to any treatment but often just stops (remits) on its own after a period of time. Most cases of migraine begin before the age of 40, so Mark's age of onset plus the constant nature of the headache from the start were strong clues that he did not have migraine. Fortunately for Mark, his headache stopped spontaneously 9 months after it began.

As you can see, things get complicated when we ask, "Do I have migraine?" Sometimes finding the answer is easy, sometimes more challenging. Box 2.4 can give you a pretty good start in making the diagnosis—though we hasten to remind you that the final diagnosis should be made by a medical specialist.

Chapter 3

The Nature and Causes of Migraine

In this chapter we consider how migraine manifests and what causes it. To get a start on thinking about these matters, let's look at a representative example:

Jerry is a 38-year-old engineer who has had headaches since his late teens. These were initially very infrequent, but they are now occurring approximately once a week. Some of these headaches are very severe; some are less so. Most of the headaches occur on both sides of his head, although some can be on just one or the other side. Many of the headaches are accompanied by nausea. Most of Jerry's headaches are easy to manage either with over-the-counter medication such as ibuprofen or by relaxing and going into a dark, quiet room. Some of the headaches can be very intrusive and debilitating, and they have, at times, caused him to miss work or at least reduce his activities during work. Jerry does not know of any other people in his family who have headaches, although all his grandparents died before he was born and his father left the family when Jerry was young, so he really doesn't know much about that side of his family. He has no siblings, and he has no other medical problems to speak of. When he first sought attention from a headache specialist he was very animated and repeatedly said, "I just want to know what's causing these headaches!"

Migraine in History

Jerry's urge to explain the cause of his headaches is very common and of course understandable. Our understanding of migraines and their causes has gone through a number of changes over the millennia. In ancient times migraines were felt to be due to divine or supernatural intervention. In some ancient cultures a severe headache was felt to be proof that an alien spirit of some sort had invaded the sufferer's head—hence the only cure would be to somehow remove it. This led people to do life-threatening drilling of holes through the skull to allow the demons to escape. This procedure is called trephination or trepanning, and ancient human skulls with holes due to trephination can still be found in archaeological digs. The amazing thing is that apparently some—though certainly not all—of the poor headache sufferers actually survived these procedures (there is evidence of wound healing in some specimens). In more recent times witchcraft was sometimes invoked as a cause, leading, as one might imagine, to equally extreme measures.

Psychological causes were also blamed for migraines and other headaches. These ideas were based not so much on evidence as on prevailing theories about poorly understood medical illnesses of the times. Unfortunately, many of these theories were so pervasive that they influenced medical thought for hundreds of years. More recently, "vascular" theories emerged for migraine mechanisms: blood vessels in the brain or scalp were thought to undergo swelling or constriction, leading to pain. This line of thought was plausible, since many migraine headaches tend to throb at around the frequency of one's heartbeat, which of course might implicate swollen or otherwise abnormal arteries. A recent study, however, revealed that the pulsations people with migraines experience do not actually happen at the rate of one's heartbeat, despite what they feel like.

Scientific Advances in Understanding Migraine

In the past 20 years or so, some firmer information has surfaced suggesting that blood vessels do in fact seem to be involved in the production of migraines—but in a different way than was imagined in the last century. It seems that the root cause of migraine pain involves *inflammation* of the blood vessels on the surface of the brain and some pain-sensitive structures near them. How this inflammation comes to occur seems to depend on a number of factors. A first step is thought to be the occurrence of an electrical wave of activity in the brain called *cortical spreading depression*. This fascinating phenomenon, which was discovered by a Brazilian neurophysiologist named Aristides Leão, seems to occur in the brains of all mammals, including humans, as a response to certain triggers. This electrical oddity seems to be very likely to occur in people who have migraine compared with those who do not. The process spreads from the back of the brain toward the front of the brain in a very slow progression, as little as approximately 1 or 2 millimeters per minute (slower than a 10th of an inch per minute). This cortical electrical wave seems to cause excitation in a part of the brain called the brainstem, which then produces changes in the branches of the trigeminal nerve that surround certain brain blood vessels. This is the link to the blood vessel inflammation that causes the pain of migraine—at least that is the current thinking. Fortunately, cortical spreading depression seems to pose no significant risk. Have a look at Fig. 3.1 for a schematic representation of the chain of events leading to migraine.

Aura

Migraine aura phenomena such as visual changes, sensation changes (tingling of the arm, face, or leg), feelings of dizziness

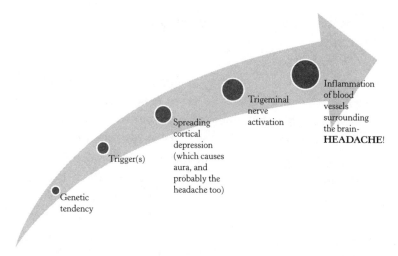

Inflammation of blood vessels surrounding the brain-**HEADACHE!**

Trigeminal nerve activation

Spreading cortical depression (which causes aura, and probably the headache too)

Trigger(s)

Genetic tendency

FIG. 3.1 The process of migraine.

and lightheadedness, and even weakness are probably manifestations of this spreading electrical phenomenon. Auras tend to occur before head pain begins, but this is not always the case; auras may occur during or after headaches.

Box 3.1 lists the kinds of migraine auras one can experience. The most common aura is the "classical" visual aura, which can consist of various changes in one's vision, including an area of grayness or even an inability to see within the entire the visual field. Sometimes the blurry areas are surrounded by bright, jagged lines or twinkling lights (see Fig. 3.2). Another visual phenomenon, which can be downright scary, is the sensation that objects are either smaller or larger than they actually are. This is called the Alice in Wonderland syndrome, since, if you recall, she got larger and smaller depending on which little pill she ate. (Don't worry; those pills are not used in headache treatment—yet.) Another manifestation in the visual realm is probably best described as "wavy vision." Some of our patients have described it as the way the air looks over

BOX 3.1 Migraine Aura Symptoms and Corresponding
Medical Terminology

Sparkling lights (scintillations)
Jagged bright lines (fortification spectra)
Wavy vision
"Holes" in vision (scotomas)
Tingling or other sensation changes (paresthesias)
Dizziness
Trouble speaking (aphasia)
Confusion, distraction
Weakness (paresis)

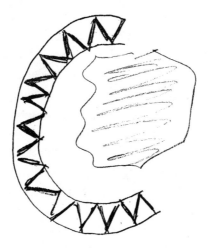

FIG. 3.2 A patient's drawing of their aura, showing the area of loss of
vision ("scotoma") surrounded by a semicircle of bright zigzag lines.

a hot barbecue grill or as resembling "heat waves" rising off pavement.

As for changes in sensation, a number of migraine sufferers experience numbness or tingling in the tips of their fingers or ends of their toes, which then begins to spread upward to sometimes include an entire half of their body, even the face. More uncomfortable and more complicated auras, which are still not very well understood, are the feelings of vertigo and lightheadedness some migraine sufferers experience. Vertigo is the sensation that either the world or oneself is moving around in a circle. This can of course be quite disturbing and disabling and can lead patients to see various specialists until it becomes clear that the symptoms might be part of their migraines. Lightheadedness is the feeling of near fainting, which many of us know as the way we sometimes feel for a few seconds after standing up too quickly. Some of our patients with this aura sensation progress to actually losing consciousness—something we are very nervous about, since it can be downright dangerous.

Another aura phenomenon is difficulty with communication, also known as *aphasia*. This can be so profound as to prevent intelligible communication. People who have this kind of aura are temporarily unable to speak, although they generally know what they would like to say and can understand all that is going on around them. Confusion can also be part of an aura. One of our patients succinctly said in frustration, "I hate how stupid I get before I get a migraine!"

Finally, people with migraine aura can experience true weakness of an arm or leg or an entire half of their body. This can look like the symptom of a stroke if there is no previous history of migraine or other clues to the fact that migraine aura is occurring. This particular type of migraine aura tends to run in families, and specific genes have been identified as causing this phenomenon.

One of the lingering questions about migraine is whether people with migraines accompanied by auras have the same condition that people with migraines without aura have. Most people who have migraine auras also have some headaches without any aura whatsoever. And in some people auras may occur without any headaches occurring at all, which makes the whole situation difficult to diagnose.

Genetics

The genetic link in the migraine story has of course been apparent to many patients and physicians because of how common migraine seems to be in certain families. In fact it is fair to say that migraine is a genetic illness. However, migraine most likely can result from different genetic abnormalities and probably is often *polygenic*, meaning that for the disorder to occur

---

BOX 3.2 Some Monogenic Causes of Migraine

- Familial hemiplegic migraine (FHM) types 1, 2, and 3
- Cerebral autosomal dominant arteriopathy with subcortical infarcts and dementia (CADASIL)
- Mitochondrial encephalomyopathy, lactic acidosis, and stroke-like episodes (MELAS); this condition is maternally inherited

in a particular individual requires multiple genetic traits. (This is true for a number of illnesses, including diabetes.) Box 3.2 lists several migraine-causing conditions that are *monogenic* (caused by a single genetic abnormality) and strongly hereditary. Of course, it is important to remember that some people with migraine may have a family history but not know about it for one reason or another.

Chapter 4

The Impact of Migraine

Migraine affects people differently at different times in their life. Disability results from the severity of the attacks, how often they occur, and how long they last. Let's first look at a few patient stories illustrating both how significantly migraine can affect the people who have it and some of the preventable causes.

Our first patient finds she cannot adequately control her headaches:

Mary has had migraines since her teenage years. She is now 37 years old. Triggers for her migraines seem to be stress and her period. Overall, she is having 8–10 headache days per month. In a typical month 3 or 4 of these attacks will be mild to moderately severe. The pain of these latter attacks, which she describes as "pressure," involves her entire head. There is nausea but no vomiting. Mary finds if she takes a 100-milligram sumatriptan (Imitrex) tablet the headache is always relieved within 1–2 hours. Unfortunately she has a second type of migraine attack, which usually awakens her the day before her menses (or sometimes on the morning her menses starts). This headache, which has a pounding feeling, involves either the right or left side of her head, and she develops nausea and vomiting quite rapidly after the attack starts. Light and sound are extremely unpleasant, and she must lie down. A sumatriptan tablet does not work. This headache can last 2–3 days. As a result, Mary misses work. Sometimes she will get a similar headache about 2 weeks after her period starts. Concerned about these more severe attacks, Mary and her husband come to the office asking what might be done about them.

Our second patient is taking more pills but experiencing more pain:

Lynda has had migraines since elementary school. They used to be infrequent, occurring about 5–6 times a year, and never lasted more than a few hours. Over-the-counter medications were always sufficient to control them, and she was never told she had migraine, although her mother had occasional "sinus headaches." Now, at age 46, she realizes her headaches have become much more frequent. For the past few weeks she has had a mild, constant background headache, which feels like pressure and sometimes is pounding. It involves her whole head. She has been using Tylenol or Excedrin to control it, taking something at least twice a day. She comes to the office worried that something serious is going on, because the pain seems to be increasing in intensity and is starting to make her feel nauseated. In the office she is a little "shaky," with a slightly rapid pulse rate of 112 beats per minute.

Finally, our third patient seems to be experiencing undesired consequences of some of his medication:

Ralph is 61-year-old man who has had frequent headaches "all my life"—by which he means since the first grade. Even then they would happen more than half the month, and he never had anything to take that reduced his headache. The headache attacks were severe and accompanied by nausea but were often relieved by vomiting. Realizing this, Ralph actually used to put his fingers down his throat to try to induce vomiting to stop the headaches. Matters changed in the 1990s, when his doctor put him on an anti-nausea drug called metoclopramide (Reglan). After this, the nature of his headache attacks changed, and if he took the metoclopramide with a pain pill such as ibuprofen, the attacks would often subside within 2–3 hours and he wouldn't vomit. He has been using this regimen to control his migraines about 20 days per month. In the past few weeks his wife has noticed some unusual movements in his face, especially around his mouth: uncontrolled and nearly constant grimacing, sometimes with blinking. Ralph was unaware of this until his wife pointed it out to him.

Disability Due to Migraine

The level of impact from migraines varies among individuals from hardly any to quite severe. Dr. Richard Lipton and his colleagues at the Montefiore Headache Center in New York have shown that as a group, migraine patients are on the lower end of the socioeconomic spectrum. We think this is because migraine can cause significant disability for many people, resulting in failure in school and in employment. Some sufferers miss school or go to school but carry on with difficulty. Work may be similarly affected; we have seen people lose their jobs because of missing work or poor performance at work related to migraine (Fig. 4.1). Migraine also of course affects family, leisure, and other social activities (Box 4.1). Many people who have the condition are not even aware of their diagnosis or do not seek out the best care. This leads them to be unnecessarily resigned to giving up many important and pleasurable activities.

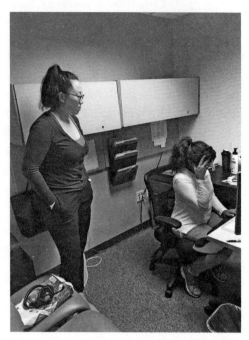

FIG. 4.1 Migraine can lead to missed days at work and at school, but just as devastating, it can cause poor performance—either of which can lead to school failure or job loss.

BOX 4.1 How Migraine Affects All Aspects of Life

- Work: absences, reduced productivity, errors, need for comprehensive medical insurance
- School: missing classes, missing assignments, poor performance on or missing exams, poor work quality
- Social life: missing important events, inability to plan for social experiences, inability to take on family or other roles
- Relationships: inability to share leisure time events, inability to take trips, sexual apathy

In our headache clinics we first make a diagnosis and make sure we are aware of any other medical conditions the patient may have. We then measure the degree of disability, sometimes by using the MIDAS (Migraine Disability Assessment Scale) test (Box 4.2). We also try hard to find out exactly how often the headache attacks occur and what the symptoms are (especially if there is nausea or vomiting). An important tool is the **headache diary** (Fig. 4.2), in which patients record headache occurrences, their severity and duration, and the treatments used, along with the response to these treatments. If a patient has more than one headache type, this can be noted too. The information from diaries gives our patients and clinicians the information they need to create reasonable goals for dealing with the patients' migraine.

Goals in Managing Migraine

When seeing a provider about your headaches it is important to choose a goal or goals for your visit and also for your long-term management. You and your provider should outline what you want to accomplish together and make a plan so that things can in fact get better (Box 4.3). There are many treatment options, and your preferences should always be taken into account. A "cookbook" approach to care is usually not a good idea; instead, an individualized treatment plan should be designed, keeping you in mind. "Treatment should not be worse than the problem" is a very good guiding principle!

One goal often chosen is to reduce the frequency and severity of migraine attacks. This brings up the topic of preventive therapies, which we will discuss in Chapters 7 and 8. Some patients do not need or want prevention, and some preventive treatments have side effects that might be undesirable. Patients want to feel well on days without a migraine and do not like to feel "medicated." A discussion about your goals and options serves to help

BOX 4.2 Migraine Disability Assessment Scale (MIDAS)

MIDAS contains the following questions:

1. On how many days in the last 3 months did you miss work or school because of your headaches?
2. How many days in the last 3 months was your productivity at work or school reduced by half or more because of your headaches? (Do not include days you counted in question 1 where you missed work or school.)
3. On how many days in the last 3 months did you not do household work because of your headaches?
4. How many days in the last 3 months was your productivity in household work reduced by half of more because of your headaches? (Do not include days you counted in question 3 where you did not do household work.)
5. On how many days in the last 3 months did you miss family, social, or leisure activities because of your headaches?

Also:

A. On how many days in the last 3 months did you have a headache? (If a headache lasted more than 1 day, count each day.)
B. On a scale of 0–10, on average how painful were these headaches (where 0 = no pain at all and 10 = pain as bad as it can be)?

Adding up all of the answers leads to a MIDAS score. Which of the following scoring categories fits you?

0–5: MIDAS grade I, little or no disability

6–10: MIDAS grade II, mild disability

11–20: MIDAS grade III, moderate disability

21 and higher: MIDAS grade IV, severe disability

Reused with permission from Walter Stewart, Richard Lipton, Andrew Dowson, and James Sawyer. Development and testing of the Migraine Disability Assessment (MIDAS) Questionnaire to assess headache-related disability. *Neurology* March 1, 2001 vol. 56 no. suppl 1 S20–S28 doi: http://dx.doi.org/10.1212/WNL.56.suppl_1.S20

Headache Log

Date	Headache severity	Duration	Meds used	Triggers	Menstrual Period
1					
2					
3					
4					
5					
6					
7					
8					
9					
10					
11					
12					
13					
14					
15					
16					
17					
18					
19					
20					
21					
22					
23					
24					
25					
26					
27					
28					
29					
30					
31					

Key:
Severity level—1–10 (1 is nearly non-existent, 10 is the worst pain you can imagine)
Medications—use abbreviations:

FIG. 4.2 An example of a monthly headache diary. Key information to note includes the occurrence, duration, and severity of migraines and what treatment the patient used. Another headache diary format can be seen in Figure 11.1.

> **BOX 4.3 Goals of Migraine Management**
>
> - Goals should be agreed upon by you and your provider
> - Management should aim for "self-efficacy" (being able to control your headaches yourself)
> - Management should include rapid, dependable relief of acute attacks
> - Side effects of treatments, both acute and preventive, should be acceptable
> - If preventive treatment is used, there should be periodic assessments to determine the need to continue, adjust, or change treatment (and to make sure it continues to be safe)
> - For headaches that don't respond to usual treatment, there should be access to rescue treatment (either self-administered or at provider's office, infusion suite, or emergency room)

you and your provider decide whether to start prevention and, if so, what treatment to choose.

Most patients will still have a need for options to treat individual attacks, which we will discuss in Chapters 5 and 6. Here too there are many choices and strategies, some quite clever. As we will discuss in those chapters, taking pills for migraine attacks with a lot of nausea or vomiting usually is not appropriate, and those attacks can be controlled in other ways.

Some Practical Examples

Let's get back to our patient case histories, thinking about them in terms of the impact headaches can make on people's lives.

Mary had migraines, of which the more severe ones were associated with her menstrual periods and sometimes with ovulation, which occurs about 2 weeks before menses (though she perceived this as headaches occurring about 2 weeks *after* her menses, as noted above). She could control her milder headaches, but the attacks with nausea and vomiting were not responding to her pills, which should not be a surprise. Her nurse practitioner wisely discussed other options for her, which included sumatriptan (Imitrex) nasal spray, sumatriptan nasal powder (Onzetra), and sumatriptan injection. Mary chose the sumatriptan nasal powder and found she could control the more severe attacks, although some days she needed a second dose, and sometimes she needed repeated treatment for 2–3 days. Her headache frequency decreased from 10 to 8 days per month, and she could control all her headaches, still using the sumatriptan pills for the milder attacks without vomiting.

Lynda actually had three problems. First, she had migraine. Second, something had made it worse: she told us she was "taking more pills and having more headaches." Third, her physician ordered a thyroid test, and it turned out she had become mildly hyperthyroid. To reassure everyone, a brain MRI was performed, the results of which were normal. Knowing that, her doctor treated her hyperthyroidism and stopped the over-the-counter medications (one of which contained caffeine). As we discussed in Chapter 1, patients who take certain medications too frequently can get a condition called medication overuse headache (analgesic rebound). This seems to be something migraine sufferers are especially prone to develop. To avoid this, many physicians try to limit use of immediate-relief migraine treatments to 2–3 days per week. With her doctor's changes, Lynda's headache frequency decreased from daily to 14 days per month. She began a preventive medication (propranolol) for her headaches and found that for acute attacks naproxen sodium (Aleve, Anaprox DS) was effective and caused her no problems.

Ralph had developed a troublesome side effect from one of his medications. Metoclopramide (Reglan) occasionally can cause a movement disorder known as tardive dyskinesia. The abnormal movements most often involve the face, though they can affect other parts of the body. Limiting the use of this agent seems prudent. In addition, Ralph, like Lynda, seemed to be suffering some degree of medication overuse headache. In retrospect, a preventive drug would have reduced his need to use acute medications to relieve headache so frequently. Using other treatments, not just pills, might also have resulted in a better outcome. When Ralph's metoclopramide and ibuprofen were stopped, his headache frequency decreased from 20 to 12 days per month. He was then put on valproate (Depakote) as a preventive medication, which reduced his headache attacks to 3–4 times a month. Sumatriptan pills and nasal sprays were quite effective in treating these. Gradually, Ralph's abnormal movements became much less noticeable.

Chapter 5

Relieving a Migraine Headache

The Best Medical Treatments

Let's look at three patients whose current migraine treatments are unsuccessful in various ways.

Paula is a 34-year-old woman who has had migraine for about 20 years. She typically will get a couple of mild-to-moderate headaches each month, which she can control with 2–3 tablets of over-the-counter ibuprofen. These headaches are not disabling; she just has mild head pressure and no other symptoms. Some months, however, she will get a much more severe headache that wakes her up 1–2 days before her period. These headaches are more than just pressure; they pound, and there is extreme nausea, which is briefly lessened when she vomits. Ibuprofen does not work for these headaches, nor do several other pills her nurse practitioner has tried. Paula misses 1–2 days of work with these headaches, and her supervisor has given her a "talking to" about this problem.

Medication hasn't worked for any of this next patient's headaches.

Tom recalls having had severe headaches since elementary school. They are infrequent (3–4 attacks yearly) but accompanied by severe nausea, vomiting, and diarrhea lasting 2–3 days. At 40 years of age this pattern remains unchanged. Pills have never helped, despite his trying many different types, and he has ended up in the emergency room when the vomiting does not stop. He has given up all hope of being helped, saying: "I've tried all the pills and they never work. My doctor doesn't know of any other treatments."

Medication is helping our last patient, but she may be overusing it.

Maria is 27 years old. Before most of her headaches, especially the severe ones, she experiences 20–30 minutes of flashing wavy lines in her vision. Sometimes she will see the lights without any headache following, but that is quite uncommon. She has learned that if she takes her pills (a triptan medication) during the aura she can often control the headache quite well. She says that while she doesn't like taking pills, her doctor is concerned that she may be using them too often. In the past she developed an ulcer from using ibuprofen "a lot."

At the end of the chapter we will see how changes in their treatment helped Paula, Tom, and Maria.

Tailoring Treatment

Basically, the way to treat a migraine attack is to give the *right dose* (usually the maximal tolerated dose) of the *right medication* at the *right time* (usually early on in the attack) by the *right route*: oral (for pills), nasal (for sprays), rectal (for suppositories), transdermal (for a skin patch), or injection. Sometimes pills are the wrong way to take migraine medicine, especially if you have a lot of nausea and vomiting.

Migraine patients may have more than one type of attack and therefore may need more than one treatment option. So the characteristics of your attacks (speed of onset of pain, nausea or vomiting, level of pain severity), your preferences, and other medical conditions you may have all may play a role in choosing how to treat your migraine headaches. Non-pharmacologic measures, acute treatment options for each headache attack, and sometimes preventive pharmacologic treatments may all be appropriate.

The most important point, however, is that treatment of migraine should be individualized. The plan should be tailored to you—"customized," so to say. A more comprehensive and personalized approach to managing migraine should result in a better outcome.

The Fundamentals

If a headache occurs, you should have a plan. Simple things like always having your medication with you are important. This means having your medication immediately accessible, not at home if you are in your office or packed away in your suitcase in the cargo hold if you are on a plane. Typically we recommend taking your headache medicine early in the attack, while the pain is still mild, if possible. You should also have a plan for what to do if the headache doesn't go away or if it comes back later. Finally, you should have a plan for what to do if matters get out of control—what we call a "rescue" plan. Rescue should include (1) something you can use as a second line for pain control,

(2) something to stop you from vomiting and enable you to get to sleep, or (3) even calling your healthcare provider for an immediate clinic visit or to be sent to the emergency room.

Choosing Treatment Options Based on Characteristics of Attacks

Box 5.1 lists several pharmacologic treatments for acute migraine attacks. Milder headaches may respond to an adequate early dose of an over-the-counter medication. This might be ibuprofen (Motrin), naproxen sodium (Aleve), or a combination medication with aspirin, acetaminophen, and caffeine (Excedrin). Sometimes we favor a prescription-strength dose of a non-steroidal anti-inflammatory drug (NSAID) such as diclofenac potassium (Cambia, Cataflam) or naproxen sodium (Anaprox). This should be taken on an empty stomach, as taking it with food will delay the effect.

BOX 5.1 Some Acute Migraine Medications

- NSAIDs such as ibuprofen (Motrin), naproxen sodium (Aleve, Anaprox), indomethacin (Indocin), and diclofenac (Cambia, Cataflam)
- Combination medicines containing butalbital, caffeine, and aspirin or acetaminophen (Fiorinal, Fioricet, Esgic) used sparingly and with caution; often cause rebound headaches and are sometimes best avoided
- Isometheptene/dichoralphenazone/acetaminophen (Midrin)

If there is nausea we may add a drug to suppress it, such as hydroxyzine (Atarax, Vistaril). Ideally this should not be taken too often (2–3 times a week at most to avoid rebound headaches). One NSAID, indomethacin (Indocin), comes as a suppository and so can be very helpful for severe headaches when vomiting is occurring; we sometimes use a suppository such as promethazine (Phenergan) in combination with indomethacin to stop vomiting. Another NSAID, ketorolac (Toradol), can be given as an intramuscular shot (we sometimes teach patients how to do this for themselves on a limited basis), and an intravenous formulation is popular for use in the emergency room. There is also a nasal spray formulation of ketorolac (Sprix).

Several medications that can be effective against migraine, including Fiorinal and Fioricet, contain the short-acting sedative butalbital. However, these can be habit-forming and can easily lead to analgesic rebound, so we rarely prescribe them. Midrin is a combination headache reliever containing a sedative as well as acetaminophen and other ingredients that sometimes works to relieve migraine pain.

If the headache pain is moderate or severe, stronger measures may be more effective. So if the pain is worsening despite early treatment or if you wake up with a headache (attacks that wake you up are usually severe), we often recommend a triptan (Box 5.2). These drugs are all available as pills, but two are also available as nasal sprays (Fig. 5.1) and one as a subcutaneous injection (Fig. 5.2); these latter choices may be better if you have nausea, vomiting, or both. Triptans have largely replaced the older class of ergot drugs (e.g., Cafergot), although some patients still use ergots, and headache experts and emergency room doctors often use dihydroergotamine (DHE-45) intravenously. DHE can also be used as a nasal spray (Migranal), and an inhaled formulation (Semprana) has been under development for some time but is not yet approved by the US Food and

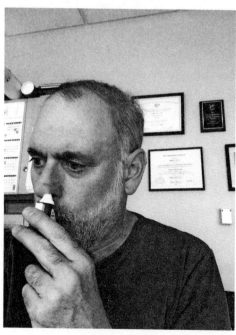

FIG. 5.1 A patient using sumatriptan in nasal spray form at the time of a migraine.

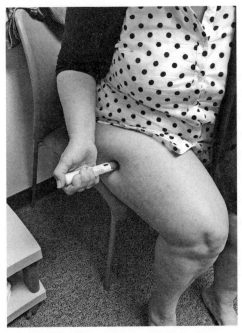

FIG. 5.2 A patient using sumatriptan in the subcutaneous (just below the surface of the skin) injectable form, which tends to be more potent and quicker acting than pills or nasal spray.

Drug Administration (FDA). DHE can also be compounded into suppositories and can be given as an intramuscular or subcutaneous injection. We sometimes teach our patients how to self-inject DHE.

Options for Recurrence and Rescue

As we have seen, there are many options to treat an acute migraine attack. Sometimes you may need to have more than one option, especially if you have more than one type of attack. If your headache recurs, simply repeating the treatment may be

---

BOX 5.3 Medications for Nausea and Vomiting

Hydroxyzine (Atarax, Vistaril): pills, capsules
Metoclopramide (Reglan): pills
Promethazine (Phenergan): pills, injection, suppositories
Prochlorperazine (Compazine): pills, suppositories, injection
Ondansetron (Zofran): pills

---

sufficient. If the first treatment fails, however, you may employ a stronger option as a backup plan; this needs to be planned with your doctor. If all these attempts fail to control the headache, then "rescue" should be employed. We use rescue measures to stop vomiting if it occurs (Box 5.3) and to allow you to get to sleep (Box 5.4). Falling into a deep sleep often will terminate a tough headache attack. Migraineurs will tell you that during an attack they desperately want such sleep but often cannot get it.

BOX 5.4 Examples of Rescue Plans

- Hydroxyzine (Vistaril) or diazepam (Valium) at a dose sufficient to allow deep sleep
- Promethazine suppositories (to stop vomiting, produce sleep, or both)
- Oral opioids (such as hydrocodone or oxycodone) used *very* sparingly
- If necessary, going to the doctor's office or emergency room for injections

---

People who have had an entrenched migraine for several days may have dozed off or slept lightly during the ordeal but probably have not really fallen into a deep, restful sleep.

If rescue measures fail, then the last resort is often to go either to the doctor's office or to the emergency room for an injection. Certainly, if there has been persistent vomiting or the headache has gone on for more than a day, it may be important to go to the emergency room or even be admitted to the hospital.

Successful Migraine Relief: Our Examples

You may now be able to imagine how the very different headache problems of the the three cases at the start of this chapter might be dealt with. Let's see what actually happened to them.

Paula usually could control her milder migraines with ibuprofen, which she did not overuse. She knew to take an adequate dose and took it early during her migraine attack. However, she had a second type of migraine that was tougher to treat. Like many adults, she got some of her headaches at night or in the early morning, and if they happened to wake her up they were already full-blown or nearly so. Migraineurs like to be able to manage their own attacks, and Paula needed a second option. Because there was nausea and vomiting, something other than a pill was the choice. In discussion with her healthcare provider Paula chose sumatriptan (Imitrex) injection. Her injection kit was set up so that she did not have to see the needle (there is even another type of injection that is "needle-free"), and she learned to inject herself if she woke up with a severe headache. After injections she felt some pressure in her throat and chest for a few minutes and has some flushing, which her provider told her are typical triptan sensations, bothersome but not threatening. After these sensations passed, she could feel her headache vanishing; typically it was gone in less than 30 minutes. If she caught it early enough, she could get back to sleep. Her provider also wisely suggested that Paula have some rescue option that she could use if the injection failed to work. They chose promethazine (Phenergan) suppositories, which are sedating and also stop vomiting. With options to deal with both of her headache types, Paula felt empowered. Because her periods were a trigger and occurred fairly regularly, Paula could be prepared for the few days during the month when she might have more severe headache. This would stop her missing work and, indirectly, lower her stress.

Tom had infrequent but severe headaches with nausea, vomiting, and diarrhea. He feared the attacks, which lasted 2–3 days. (This fear has been termed "cephalalgiaphobia," from Greek roots meaning "fear of headache.") Many different types of pills failed to relieve his headaches, and he clearly also needed a non-oral way to take his headache medicine. His provider suggested trying DHE nasal spray, but Tom found it was unreliable; it worked only for about half of his attacks. He then learned to give himself intramuscular injections of DHE (plus an oral anti-nauseant, hydroxyzine). This turned out to control all of his headaches. The DHE took 1–2 hours to fully "kick in" and had to be injected daily for 2–3 days, but Tom was much more functional during the attacks, with minimal disability and requiring no further trips to the emergency room. His doctor also gave him promethazine—taken via injection as well, because of his diarrhea—as a rescue.

Maria presented an interesting paradox. She said she did not like to take pills but overused a number of relatively ineffective treatments that happened to be pills! Patients should not take medications that don't work well if they have given those medications a fair chance. Otherwise side effects are more likely and benefits are unlikely. Some people relate that migraines that follow an aura are likely to be particularly severe. Maria's strategy of taking her triptan pill during the aura was sound and it often worked well. Unfortunately, she, like Tom, hated her migraines and had considerable anxiety about them, so she often took medication first thing in the morning as a preventive measure (she called it a "pre-emptive strike") even though her pills are designed to treat, not prevent, an attack. Her provider sent her to a psychologist for some non-pharmacologic measures to help her deal with her headaches and anxiety. She learned bio-feedback, which she began using daily. Her headache frequency declined, and she was able to use her pills only when an attack was beginning. So Maria was pleased: she had fewer headaches and could use fewer pills.

In considering options for controlling your migraine attacks, you and your provider need to consider what has worked for you in the past, what has not worked, and perhaps why it hasn't worked, and then choose treatments that take into account the nature of your headache attacks, such as whether there is vomiting during some of them. Making plans to deal with recurrence of an attack after treatment is reassuring and empowering, as is having rescue options for attacks that are unresponsive to the usual treatments.

Chapter 6

Relieving a Migraine Headache

Non-medicinal Approaches

Here is someone who really wants (and deserves to have) a reliable way out of her severe migraines:

Margaret is an administrative assistant to the CEO of a high-tech company in a large city. She works long hours, but loves her job and is highly regarded there. She gets severe headaches about once a month or, when she is lucky, once every 2 months. But these are headaches she rates "11 on a scale of 10," and she dreads them. They are often preceded by flickering "circles in my vision" that are generally perceived in her peripheral vision on one side and last about 20–30 minutes. As the circles begin to fade Margaret is able to see to do her work again but usually begins to notice a more and more severe headache on the side of her head or in her temples. This soon leads to nausea and she has to find a bathroom quickly, since she will almost always vomit once or twice. The headache is usually gone by the next morning, but the day is generally "ruined." This hurts her otherwise flawless performance at work, and she becomes teary whenever she tells her close friends about it. She learned that her mother and two of her mother's sisters all had similar headaches. She has tried a number of medications at the time of her headaches, including over-the-counter painkillers,

Fioricet, triptans, and even Percocet, but none has helped appreciably. "I just have to let it run its course," Margaret says, "but what I really need is 'a magic bullet,' and I don't want to pop pills." So far, her best option is to use 2 Excedrin tablets and a strong cup of coffee, close her door, and turn off the lights.

Like Margaret, many patients do not have success with medicinal approaches to relieving their migraine attacks or simply do not want to use such approaches. In addition to the nearly universally useful migraine strategy of rest in darkness and quiet, there are a number of other non-medicinal approaches to a migraine, which we will share in this chapter. None have been satisfactorily proven to work across a wide range of patients, but we have included all the approaches that we have found useful for selected patients to supply you with options.

Acting on Warnings of an Impending Attack

As all migraine sufferers know, the first step in relieving the pain of migraine is to find a dark, quiet place to lie down. But how can you make this first move efficiently at the workplace, at school, or in a social setting? Many migraineurs find it helpful to pay attention to any aura symptoms (visual manifestations, sensation changes, confusion, or other events that predict migraine) that usually indicate an oncoming migraine. Another group of symptoms warning of migraine but not officially constituting aura are called prodromal symptoms. These include changes in mood such as irritability, mild confusion, yawning, abdominal changes (even including the urge to defecate), and intensification of smell, brightness, and sound. If auras or prodromal symptoms are present, it is time to start any and all strategies that have helped your headaches in the past.

Simple Physical Measures

Applying cold to the head has long been a common method of combatting the initial attack of a migraine. Using a bag of frozen peas is a nice option, since one can mold the bag to the back of the head or the forehead. It is important not to leave the cold pack on your skin for too long, as it could damage the skin. A good rule of thumb is "10 minutes on, 10 minutes off."

Applying mild pressure on the head can also be helpful, and any review or Web-based search of migraine treatments will present all sorts of headbands and other means of putting a bit of pressure on the head during a migraine. The best spots tend to be the temples and just below the base of the skull. Acupuncturists have adapted their techniques to develop specific "acupressure" points that are said to help reduce the pain of migraine headaches. Fig. 6.1 shows some of the most useful of these pressure points. Also, mild pressure in the back of the head, just below the base of the skull, can help. We have also read and heard of patients obtaining relief from warming their hands with mildly hot water for several minutes.

Caffeine, Aromatherapy, and Herbal Approaches

Sometimes caffeine, in the form of coffee or tea, is helpful at the beginning of a migraine. The caffeine content in coffee varies between about 50 and 200 milligrams (mg) per cup (depending on cup size, of course). Tea has less caffeine, but a strong cup of

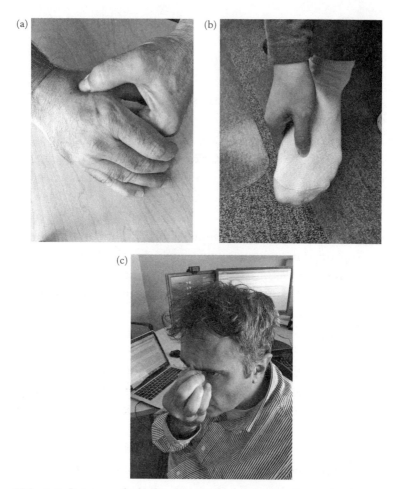

FIG. 6.1 Points on the body where acupressure can relieve migraine include (a) the area between the thumb and index finger, (b) the area between the first two toes, and (c) the bridge of the nose.

black tea might have as much as 50 mg (green tea has about half as much). Like other migraine relievers, however, caffeine can actually promote headaches when it is overused. We generally tell our patients to limit their intake to about 100 mg of caffeine per day at most and not to vary their intake much.

In many parts of the world, inhaling aromatic substances has been popular as an acute treatment for migraine for many centuries. One such treatment is "tiger balm," which contains a mixture of camphor, menthol, cajuput oil, and eucalyptus oil; other ingredients are added to some brands. It is said to work best when applied to the temples, but our feeling is that the particular location is not very important, because we believe these kinds of treatments work via a form of aromatherapy, inducing changes in the migraine process by stimulating the olfactory (smell) system in the brain. There is no strong evidence that tiger balm is effective, but many patients report finding it moderately helpful. Other aromatherapy agents have been proposed as useful against migraine, including lavender and peppermint.

A number of herbal therapies have been proposed for the relief of migraine, but most are disappointing when used acutely. Feverfew leaves have helped some patients when chewed and swallowed or taken in pill form (generally dried, powdered leaves in capsules). These leaves contain aspirin-like substances, and presumably that is how they help. It is also a reason to be careful not to overuse feverfew, the dose of which should probably not exceed 1 leaf 3 times daily. One herbal treatment, while not terribly useful for migraine headache, is quite effective for the nausea that accompanies migraine in many people: ginger. It can be used in the candied (sugared) form, pickled, or even as dried powder in capsule. It is not surprising that the candied version is most palatable—and it seems fair that there ought to be something sweet for the individual suffering from a migraine!

Magnesium has also been helpful at the time of headache for some individuals and is relatively harmless at a dose of 100–200 mg.

Many famous physicians in history, including William Osler in the late 19th century, recommended marijuana for acute relief of migraine; indeed, this was the treatment of choice of most physicians of Osler's time. Marijuana also seems to control nausea associated with migraine. The problem with marijuana, other than the lack of any real evidence for its benefits in migraine, is that it produces a mental state change that many patients do not desire. And of course before you try any cannabis product, we urge you to discuss it with your doctor and to thoroughly acquaint yourself with all legal restrictions governing the use of cannabis products in your state or country.

Behavioral Medicine Techniques

Finally, a number of what we tend to refer to as relaxation techniques may be useful for migraine relief. It seems, although again clear evidence is lacking, that if you can induce a state of deep relaxation, pain diminishes. Options include progressive muscle relaxation, biofeedback, self-hypnosis, and meditation. These all require some training but can be learned by virtually anyone, including most adolescents and children. We will go into these techniques a bit more deeply in Chapter 8, on non-medicinal preventive treatment of migraine.

Chapter 7

Preventing Migraine

Medical Choices

Not all migraineurs require preventive treatment. Frankly, treatments for an individual headache attack are much better than the preventive (prophylactic) options. There are, however, many people whose headaches cause enough disability that some form of prevention is warranted. The purpose of preventive treatments is to make the headaches fewer, milder, or briefer. Reasons to consider daily preventive medication might include (1) a high frequency of migraine attacks, (2) a high level of severity of migraine even though perhaps not so frequent, (3) high disability at one's job or school or even threat of being fired or expelled, (4) failure to respond to acute medications, and (5) intolerability of acute medications (due to medical risks or side effects).

How to Choose Preventive Medication

There are many medicinal (pharmacologic) options for preventing migraines. Chapter 8 will discuss non-pharmacologic approaches for migraine prevention, but these don't always work; sometimes, pharmacologic intervention is the only choice. The two types of approaches are not mutually exclusive. In fact the evidence suggests they are complementary, and that people who use both pharmacologic and non-pharmacologic approaches may do better than those who do not. Suffice it to say, avoiding triggers to whatever extent possible makes sense, and being regular in your habits (e.g., with respect to sleep and eating) is also helpful. But triggers are often hard to avoid, and a more aggressive approach to preventing migraines is sometimes necessary.

If you choose to try pharmacologic headache prevention, you will need a careful and thorough assessment by your medical provider. Any other medical conditions you have need to be taken into consideration when choosing a medication. Try to get a "twofer" where using one medication may not only improve your headache pattern but also help with another medical condition (see Table 7.1). It is important not to choose options that could *worsen* another medical condition you have, which is why it is essential to discuss all options with your doctor and not to make decisions on your own. The American Headache Society and the American Academy of Neurology have jointly published

TABLE 7.1 Added Benefits and Undesired Effects of Some Migraine Preventive Drugs for Other Medical Conditions

Drug	Also Helps with	May Worsen
Propranolol (Inderal)	High blood pressure, tremor, anxiety	Low blood pressure, asthma, cold extremities, depression
Verapamil (Calan)	High blood pressure, cold extremities	Irritable bowel, constipation
Valproate (Depakote)	Bipolar disorder, seizures	Overweight, tremor
Topiramate (Topamax)	Seizures, obesity	Kidney stones
Candesartan (Atacand)	High blood pressure	

evidence-based guidelines for migraine prevention in adults and children at www.aan.com. These guidelines can help you and your provider tailor a prophylactic medication regimen for you.

Let's look at several real case histories as examples of how to choose a preventive therapy for migraine.

Jonathan is a 30-year-old attorney. Both his parents have migraine, so it is not surprising that he inherited the condition. He has mild high blood pressure and asthma, which is under good control because he has given up smoking. Rizatriptan (Maxalt) has been effective for his migraine attacks, but he needs to use it 10–12 days per month. He has the impression that the number of headaches he is having monthly has been slowly increasing. Also, the rizatriptan takes nearly 2 hours to fully work, and he has had some difficulty representing his clients during that time. He would like to have fewer headaches and for the medication to work better.

Our second patient struggles with a high headache frequency, which is now seriously affecting her career.

Kim is a 61-year-old administrative assistant whose headache frequency has slowly increased over the years, from 3–4 times a month in her teens to the point where she now has nearly daily, unremitting headache. She is missing a lot of work, and her supervisor has already spoken to her the problem. When she is at work she is often carrying on with difficulty because of her headaches. Her primary care provider became concerned and ordered some tests, the results of which were reassuringly normal. Her insurance allows her only 9 sumatriptan (Imitrex) tablets a month, and she runs out of them within a week. She therefore is using acetaminophen/aspirin/caffeine (Excedrin) on a near daily basis. She knows she is using more pills and having more headaches. She has recently tried several preventive drugs that her doctor suggested, including propranolol (Inderal), which worsened the depression she was already suffering from; amitriptyline (Elavil), which made her gain 20 pounds; and valproate (Depakote), which made her shake and caused hair loss and a 30-pound weight gain. She then tried topiramate (Topamax), a drug her doctor told her might help her lose weight. In fact she lost 10 pounds, but she became, as she described it, "confused" and started making errors at work. Kim is feeling desperate and unsure what to do next.

Our last patient is looking for ways to get control over her headache pattern.

Mary Ellen is a divorced 47-year-old woman who started having migraines when she was 32 years old, at the time of the birth of her son. She finds that lack of sleep is a migraine trigger, as are certain foods (aged cheeses and red wine). Her headache frequency varies considerably month to month, depending on her sleep pattern and whether or not she is under a lot of "stress." After keeping headache calendars on her smartphone for 3 months, she finds she is averaging 6–10 days of migraine per month, with 5–6 days on a "good month" and 10 or so days during a "bad month." Mary Ellen is missing a lot of work as well as family activities.

Jonathan, Kim, and Mary Ellen each eventually found solutions for their headache problems, but they were all different. We will come back to their cases at the end of the chapter.

Options for Preventive Medication

Choosing a preventive drug therapy requires both knowledge and a bit of "art" (as you will see in the solutions arrived at for our three cases). To re-emphasize what we have said earlier, before embarking on treatment to prevent migraine, you must talk with your provider and determine what *your* goals for therapy are. Also, it is crucial to bear in mind that "prevention" does not mean your headaches will absolutely stop. More likely they will become fewer, milder, or shorter (or some combination of these).

Bearing these considerations in mind, there are a number of good options in preventive medications. Box 7.1 lists those with the best scientific evidence for their efficacy, and Box 7.2 list a number of medications that are commonly used but have somewhat less evidence to support them. People are generally surprised by how many medications developed for other illnesses

---

BOX 7.1 Migraine Preventives with Best Evidence of Efficacy

Propranolol (Inderal)

Topiramate (Topamax)

Divalproex sodium, valproate (Depakote)

Metoprolol (Lopressor)

Timolol (Blocadren)

Frovatriptan (Frova) (for short-term prophylaxis of menstrually related migraine)

OnabotulinumtoxinA (Botox) (for chronic migraine)

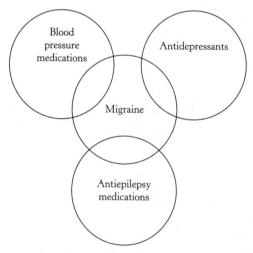

FIG. 7.1 Overlapping treatment options. Many medications developed to treat other conditions have been found to help migraine, for generally unclear reasons.

seem to help prevent migraines (see Fig. 7.1). Let's delve a little further into the main categories of these medications.

Beta Blockers

One of the oldest categories of migraine preventive medicines is the beta blockers. The best-known one is propranolol (Inderal). Most often used for control of high blood pressure, this drug has also been used for other medical conditions, including angina, tremor, and stage fright or anxiety. Back in the 1960s, during a drug study of patients with angina (chest pain), it was serendipitously noted that a patient with migraine had improvement in his headaches while taking propranolol. Sure enough, this drug and other beta blockers can be effective migraine preventives.

A beta blocker might be a good type of drug to choose if you also have high blood pressure; angina or coronary artery disease; tremor; or anxiety. These drugs, however, may worsen depression, low blood pressure, asthma, and Raynaud's phenomenon (vasospasm resulting in cold extremities or poor circulation), a condition that occurs commonly in migraineurs. They may also cause weight gain if the patient's tolerance for exercise goes down. (Box 7.3 summarizes potential side effects of migraine preventive medications, most of which tend to be minor at modest medication doses.)

Antidepressants

Depression and anxiety are often "co-morbid" with migraine; that is, the conditions often occur together. Some older antidepressants (the heterocyclic agents) have been effective for migraine prevention, of which the best studied is amitriptyline (Elavil). The very high doses sometimes necessary to treat depression have many side effects, but much lower doses can be used for migraine

---

BOX 7.3 Common Side Effects of Migraine
Preventive Drugs

Weight gain: divalproex sodium, amitriptyline,
cyproheptadine
Sedation: amitriptyline, gabapentin, cyproheptadine
Fatigue: propranolol and other beta blockers
Low blood pressure: all blood pressure medications, beta
blockers
Weight loss: topiramate, zonisamide
Clouded thinking: topiramate, gabapentin, zonisamide

---

prevention. A single dose at bedtime usually is sufficient and convenient. Bedtime dosing is used because most medications in this category are sedating and so can help insomnia as well. Side effects include tremor, weight gain, and dry mouth.

When the newer selective serotonin reuptake inhibitor (SSRI) antidepressant drugs appeared—fluoxetine (Prozac) was the first—clinicians thought they might be effective migraine treatments too, but this turned out not to be the case. An exception is a drug from a related category, a serotonin–norepinephrine reuptake inhibitor (SNRI) known as venlafaxine (Effexor). If a migraine patient has significant depression, this drug may be a very useful option for treating both conditions with one agent.

Anti-seizure Medications

Certain anticonvulsants have shown benefit in preventing migraine. The two that have the best evidence of working are topiramate (Topamax) and valproate (Depakote). Both of these drugs are approved by the FDA for preventing episodic migraine (headache occurring less than 15 days per month); additionally, topiramate has good evidence that it may work in chronic migraine (headache 15 days or more per month).

Topiramate has been used for migraine prevention at lower daily total doses than when it is used for seizure prevention. The typical target dose is about 100 mg per day, but most patients are gradually increased up to that dose; some patients may require a little less or a little more. Because this drug affects your acid–base balance, a common side effect is tingling in the hands and feet. Usually this effect is mild, but occasionally it is quite bothersome. When that is the case, the antidote is potassium (which can be gotten from potassium-rich foods like bananas and tomatoes). Other side effects include cognitive difficulties (often word-finding trouble), precipitation of kidney stones (rarely), and acute glaucoma (quite rare). Unlike many other migraine preventives, topiramate typically does not cause weight gain. In fact some patients lose weight when taking it. Higher doses (200 mg daily or more) can neutralize the effect of birth control pills.

Valproate can be a very powerful migraine preventive. It can also be associated with significant weight gain, tremor, and hair loss. Unlike topiramate, it does not interact with birth control. However, it is associated with a significant risk of the birth defect spina bifida if taken during pregnancy and is best avoided in women who may become pregnant. Many clinicians avoid this drug entirely in women, especially if they can become pregnant.

Other Preventives

In addition to beta blockers, other blood pressure medications, such as angiotensin-converting enzyme (ACE) inhibitors like lisinopril and angiotensin receptor blockers (ARBs) like candesartan, have some evidence of being helpful in preventing migraine and are often very well tolerated. Calcium channel blockers (verapamil and others) are often used as migraine preventive agents. With the exception of flunarizine, a calcium channel drug not approved in the United States, they have less evidence of being effective than other blood pressure medications. Calcium channel blockers dilate blood vessels and can improve circulation in patients with Raynaud's phenomenon. In contrast to the mixed usefulness of calcium channel blockers for preventing migraine, verapamil is the most effective drug for preventing cluster headache.

Cyproheptadine (Periactin) is a very old drug with little evidence to support its use for migraine but is very safe and often used to prevent migraine in children. It also treats allergic rhinitis. Typically taken three times a day in children, cyproheptadine can be very helpful, but it is sedating and sometimes causes impressive weight gain. For adults we have found it is useful when taken as a single night-time dose to improve sleep and suppress nightmares if they are a problem (as in some of our patients with post-traumatic stress disorder, or PTSD).

Chronic migraine (discussed in detail in Chapter 11) is of course a particularly troublesome form of migraine. The evidence suggests that two possible treatments are the most likely to work in preventing it. One is topiramate, which we have already discussed. The other is onabotulinumtoxinA (Botox). Botox in fact is the *only* FDA-approved treatment for chronic migraine. Interestingly, it does not seem to help prevent migraines in people with episodic migraine. We will talk more about it in Chapter 11.

Caution Regarding Pregnancy

We have already discussed the risks of valproate in women who might become pregnant. However, we generally avoid using *any* migraine preventive drugs in pregnancy unless absolutely necessary. We discuss contraceptive measures with our patients, because pregnancies are often unplanned, and we particularly tend to avoid those preventive drugs with riskier birth defect profiles (such as valproate) in our female patients of reproductive age. It is also advisable for patients to discuss these issues as well as their birth control with their ob-gyn providers, and for the doctors treating patients' headaches also to work closely with those providers.

Successful Medicinal Migraine Prevention: Our Examples

Let's see what was done preventively to help the headache situations of the three migraineurs discussed earlier in the chapter.

Jonathan was having more headaches per month than he or his doctor wanted. The doctor also suspected that the amount of rizatriptan Jonathan was using to treat his headaches was a little excessive and might actually have been contributing to his increasing number of attacks. Ordinarily she would have offered him prevention with propranolol to also control his high blood pressure, but that drug can worsen asthma, which Jonathan had a history of. Instead, she chose lisinopril, which treats blood pressure and might prevent migraine attacks. After 3 months on this new drug, Jonathan was having only 2–3 migraines a month and found his rizatriptan seemed to work faster when he did need it.

Kim's problem was a bit more complicated. She had worsened from episodic to chronic migraine. This might have been due to medication overuse headache, which often occurs in migraineurs who are overusing short-acting headache medications like some of the triptans (in Kim's case, sumatriptan) and combination analgesics such as Excedrin. Many preventive treatments fail to work if there is ongoing analgesic rebound. With so many treatments having failed, Kim's nurse practitioner sent her to a headache clinic. The doctor there decided she had chronic migraine with medication overuse headache. Kim was admitted to the hospital for 3 days, her sumatriptan and Excedrin were stopped, and she was treated with intravenous medication, including dihydroergotamine (DHE-45). On the second day she became headache free. She was discharged on onabotulinumtoxinA (Botox) for prevention, naproxen sodium for her milder headaches, and intranasal DHE (Migranal) for severe migraines. Kim now has about 15 headache-free days per month and is able to control what headaches she does get. Her job is no longer in jeopardy.

Mary Ellen found an easy solution to her problem. Like many migraineurs, she was never a "good sleeper." After her divorce, she found she was under more financial stress and would lie awake at night worrying. Her headache frequency increased in response. She and her provider chose amitriptyline for prevention. On just 10 mg nightly, her sleep improved from 3–4 hours a night to 6–7 hours. Her monthly headache frequency decreased to 3–4 attacks. She uses either naproxen sodium or sumatriptan to successfully manage all the attacks she gets.

It is important that the approach to managing headaches be comprehensive—by this we mean searching for the best preventive *and* migraine-relieving medications as well as non-medicinal approaches. But what may be even more important is to make sure we individualize headache management. People with migraine all differ, and treatment programs must take these differences into account.

Chapter 8

Preventing Migraine

Non-medicinal and Alternative Approaches

Over the many years that we have cared for migraine sufferers, we have commonly heard the complaint that we focus too often on pharmaceutical approaches to their headaches. This criticism is sometimes well founded. There are many effective botanical, physical, nutritional, and other non-medicinal approaches to reducing the impact of migraine. In Chapter 6 we presented non-medicinal remedies for use at the time of headache. In this chapter we will explore non-medicinal approaches to preventing migraine, a far more powerful approach (if it works) than waiting for the migraine to start before instituting treatment.

Here is the story of a person who was literally begging us to find something that would reduce the frequency of her headaches but that would not cause any of the nasty side effects that seemed to happen with all the daily preventive medications other physicians had prescribed:

Mary looked uncomfortable and unhappy when she was seen for the second time in our headache center. She blurted out: "You doctors are all the same! All you do is hand out prescriptions for pills that make me sicker than I was to start with! All the antidepressants made me gain all this weight and feel weird. In fact they *made* me depressed! The beta blockers made me tired and so did the calcium channel

blockers. Are they the same thing, by the way? The topiramate made me *stupid*, although I liked that it made me lose
a few of the pounds that I gained on the antidepressants.
The valproate made me sick and also made me gain weight!
And you won't let me take painkillers very often! I heard you
were really good—but you are just like all the other doctors
I have seen, who seemed to want to kill me. And I told you all
how sensitive to medication I am! You've run all your tests
and you all say I have migraine. But what are you going to
do about it?"

We physicians are human too, and this kind of tirade is of
course upsetting to us. However, the truth in what Mary was
telling us was powerful: she found the medications to be worse
than the disease. We are usually able to find well-tolerated medications for our patients, but searching for them can be a frustrating process for some. Luckily there are some non-medicinal
approaches that can help.

Herbal Treatments

Even though many of our pharmaceutical treatments are
derived from or inspired by botanical sources, health profession-
als in developed countries have far less commonly advocated
for herbal treatments, particularly for headaches. This seems
to be changing to some extent; certainly, many people in the
developed world use these remedies, although their healthcare
providers may not be aware of it. In Germany and France, for
example, more than half of physicians routinely prescribe herbal
medicines, and in the United States many are reaching out to
find non-pharmaceutical options for their patients who cannot
tolerate or simply prefer a non-pharmaceutical path.

Herbal therapy can be divided into three categories: oral, or "nutraceutical" (from *nutrition* plus *pharmaceutical*), therapy; topical preparations (ointments, etc.); and inhalation of various substances. There is some overlap between these categories. For example, the camphor/menthol topical creams discussed in Chapter 6 may very well work not via skin absorption but rather by the effects of their strong scents.

Scientific evidence for the efficacy of herbal medications is sparse, for a number of reasons. First, research is hard to start up: doing comparative scientific studies is expensive, and there is not a lot of funding available (nor money to be made) in alternative medicine. In addition, it is hard to quantify herbal substances and to know which strains are the most effective. The form (e.g., raw, dried, distilled) may matter, and the beneficial dose may vary significantly among individuals. Safety concerns may be less well characterized than with pharmaceuticals. In the United States, unlike some other countries, the manufacture of these non-prescription remedies is not supervised by the government, and their content and purity are therefore uncertain.

Feverfew, which we mentioned in Chapter 6, seems to be of help in preventing migraine when taken daily, either as whole leaves or dried desiccated leaf. However, it has some potential side effects, including joint aches, gastrointestinal disturbances, and mouth ulcers. Drugs that interact with feverfew include anticoagulants like warfarin (Coumadin).

Butterbur (*Petasites hybridus*) root has been shown to be effective in preventing migraine. However, it has been linked to liver cancer and other liver damage (hepatitis) if not processed properly, and because of this, fewer headache specialists now recommend it.

Chamomile, a relative of feverfew, when used as an oil derived from the flowers, seems to be effective in preventing nausea. While scientific evidence for this effect is not available, chamomile has been used for this purpose in this form, as well as in teas, in many cultures throughout history.

The tea or infusions made from the leaves of passionflower are said to be helpful in preventing headaches, but no clear evidence exists for this effect. Other nutraceuticals for which anti-headache claims have been made include valerian root, stinging nettle, juniper, peppermint, kudzu, willow, and birch. Like feverfew, the bark of willow and birch has salicylates—the same type of chemical as the active ingredient in aspirin—and we assume this underlies its mechanism of action.

Homeopathy, which essentially consists of sublingual (under the tongue) administration of highly diluted compounds derived from botanical, mineral, and other sources, does not really qualify as herbal treatment, and it defies scientific principles. Yet some patients report success using it, and it is probably entirely harmless.

Physical Exercise

There is some evidence that regular exercise prevents migraines. This surprises some of our patients, who have observed that exercise can sometimes induce a migraine. We commonly recommend moderate exercise at least 3 times weekly to our patients, but we make sure to warn them that exercise intensity should be matched to their level of conditioning (in other words, don't overdo it).

Manual Techniques

Massage on a regular basis helps many of our patients. The efficacy of massage is extremely hard to look into scientifically, as there are many massage styles and there are probably many differences in response to massage from patient to patient. Chiropractic manipulation has helped some patients, but we rarely recommend it, because (1) we have rarely seen long-lasting results from chiropractic and (2) it probably poses some risk of damage to the spine and to the blood vessels that run alongside it.

Nutritional Intervention

Look at any headache or migraine website and you will likely discover a list of "food triggers" or a description of a "migraine diet." However, we have rarely seen any standardized diet work to prevent migraine and suspect that if there are dietary strategies, they are unique to certain individuals. With gluten-free diets gaining popularity, many migraine sufferers wonder if they will benefit from them. They probably need not pursue this possibility unless they have been conclusively diagnosed with celiac disease by a knowledgeable physician.

However, there are substances that can clearly lead to migraine in some people, including alcohol; monosodium glutamate (MSG) and other food additives; histamines; nitrites and nitrates; and possibly tyramine. Alcohol is probably tolerated well by some migraineurs and not well at all by others—and they know who they are, because migraine either happens pretty quickly after consuming alcohol or occurs the next morning as part of the hangover. We tell our patients who wish to drink to do so in moderation and to avoid whichever forms of alcohol seem to be triggers for them. It is our impression that white wine, beer, and clear liquor are less productive of migraine than red wine and darker liquors. It was thought in the past that sulfites in wine led to migraine, but this has largely been debunked. The high levels of histamine in some wines may be the factor responsible for migraines, but this is not yet clear.

Foods with nitrites and nitrates including hot dogs and processed meat, are probably capable of inducing migraine, but again this is not yet clear. MSG has been shown to cause migraine-like headaches and should be avoided. It can be found in some restaurant food and is definitely present in lots of prepared canned and frozen foods, since it is a flavor preservative. It masquerades under many names, so merely looking for "MSG" or "monosodium glutamate" on a list of ingredients may not be sufficient (see Box 8.1).

BOX 8.1 Some Aliases for Monosodium Glutamate

Autolyzed yeast
Hydrolyzed cornstarch
Hydrolyzed gelatin
Hydrolyzed milk protein
Hydrolyzed plant protein
Hydrolyzed protein
Hydrolyzed soy
Hydrolyzed wheat
Hydrolyzed yeast
MSG
Partially hydrolyzed protein
Plant protein extract
Textured protein
Yeast extract

Dietary Supplements

In addition to herbal remedies, a number of other naturally occurring substances have been promoted for use in preventing migraine in recent years, including vitamins and other nutraceuticals. Those with the best evidence of efficacy include magnesium (in chelated forms such as magnesium gluconate and magnesium taurate) and riboflavin (vitamin B2). The useful daily dose of magnesium seems to be in the 500- to 600-mg range. Magnesium can cause loose stools and so may be a problem for some people. Riboflavin is essentially free of side effects and, in a dose of around 400 mg daily, seems effective in reducing migraine frequency and severity for some patients. Another supplement, coenzyme Q10 (CoQ10), seems to be helpful at a dose of 150–300 mg daily for many patients as well. Other supplements, such as S-adenosyl methionine (SAM-e) and other amino acid–derived substances, have little or no evidence supporting their use.

Meditation and Relaxation Approaches

More than 50 years ago a Harvard Medical School professor, Herbert Benson, developed the idea that some illnesses were worsened by what he called the "stress response," also known as the "fight or flight" response. The fight-or-flight state is an intense physiological condition our bodies get into when we feel physically or emotionally threatened. We all know it well, having experienced it many times in our lives. A speedy heart rate, sweating, tensing of muscles, rapid breathing—these are all familiar manifestations of the response. There are unconscious manifestations too, also designed to help us evade danger and protect ourselves when threatened. The problem is that our bodies are programmed to sometimes go into a stressed state even when it is not helpful—and even in some situations where it is actually bad for us. Benson's work led a generation of investigators to explore the possibility that if we can prevent the stress response and enter a relaxed state, we can become healthier and happier. Benson's book *The Relaxation Response* became a bestseller in the 1970s, and it continues to be popular.

Many approaches have been proposed for attaining this relaxed state, with the assumption that if we can "turn it on" we can avert medical consequences of stress such as high blood pressure, ulcers, asthma, bladder problems, muscle tension, and, yes, migraine. Whether this assumption is universally true is not yet known. It may be that for some people, preventing the stress response is life-saving, but for others is not particularly potent medically. On the other hand, most people want to gain some control over their reactions to threatening situations, so we feel that training in achieving relaxed states is almost always well worth the effort.

Popular approaches to achieving a relaxed mental state include biofeedback, meditation, hypnosis, yoga, and many others. Biofeedback refers to a set of techniques that show people how their bodies are functioning and simultaneously teach them how to alter some of those unconscious states (Fig. 8.1). For example, in "hand-warming" (thermal-guided) biofeedback, a computer screen or other device shows how warm or cold one's hand is becoming during certain activities. The biofeedback student then learns some maneuvers and tricks to warm the hands without any external source of heat. These hand-warming techniques are, to put it simply, learned skills for changing blood flow. If you can warm your hands using your mind, you are actually affecting the parts of the autonomic nervous system that control blood vessels. If the arteries constrict, as is common in the fight-or-flight state, your hands become cold. If the arteries

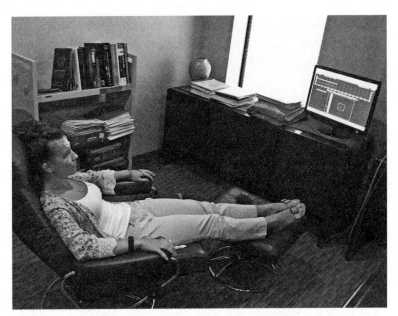

FIG. 8.1 A patient practicing biofeedback. She practices certain mental exercises while receiving feedback about her success in producing a relaxed state. (Photograph used by permission from Dr. Steven Baskin and Dr. Randall Weeks, New England Institute for Neurology and Headache, Stamford, CT.)

dilate, more blood flows and the extremities become warmer. The idea is that if you can warm your hands mentally, you can reverse the stress response. Similar methods have been proposed for learning how to watch your brainwaves and change them or to watch a readout of the muscle tension, say, in your neck and reduce it using only your mind. Such techniques may sound like magic, but they have been shown many times to be learnable.

Meditation also aims to achieve a relaxed state that is virtually the opposite of the stress response. But more than that, as meditators can attest, regular meditation can produce a lasting lower baseline level of physiological excitement when you don't want it. There are a number of forms of meditation across the world, done in different positions and taught in different ways, but they seem to produce the same sort of beneficial physical effects.

Hypnosis is another means of entering a state similar to the meditative state for the purposes of improving headache pain and suffering. It is best taught in the form of self-hypnosis. Here an experienced hypnotherapist finds a way that lets the learner most quickly enter the trance state and then helps the learner practice until that state is easier and easier to achieve. Hypnosis has other purposes, such as reducing anxiety and instilling motivation to stop smoking or overeating, but one thing it is *not* is some devious form of mind control as depicted in certain movies. People in a hypnotic trance can leave it at will any time they like, and no one has ever committed an act during a trance that he or she normally would be unwilling to do.

Successful Non-medicinal Migraine Prevention: An Example

Let's return to Mary's predicament. Luckily we were able to help her using some of the ideas discussed above.

At the end of the follow-up visit described at the start of this chapter, Mary burst into tears. Her headache diary showed approximately 4 headache days per week and 6–8 severe migraines every month. She was using some kind of painkiller on most days, generally an over-the-counter medicine like ibuprofen or acetaminophen. We gave her a mild analgesic that rarely causes medication overuse headache and told her to absolutely limit her use of stronger medications for relief to 2 days per week. Because her weight was really upsetting her, we shared with her how important exercise and diet were in controlling migraine. We discussed exercise types she liked, and she constructed a weekly schedule showing exactly when she would carve out time for exercise. Our nurse spent time with her outlining a new diet emphasizing regular mealtimes, perhaps a bit more frequent than before but with smaller portions, low sugar, no additives, no alcohol, one small serving of caffeine per day, and good hydration. She was told to start taking magnesium preventively, and we talked about ginger as an anti-nauseant. We scheduled an appointment for biofeedback to help her learn how to achieve the "relaxation response."

At her next visit, Mary seemed much happier, which she explained was because she didn't have a headache that day. She said she was doing all the things we advised and had lost 12 pounds in the 2-month interval but was still having "lots of headaches." When we looked at her headache log, she saw to her surprise that over the last 2 months she had had about the same number of headaches she used to have in 1 month. At the next visit these numbers had dropped even further.

Mary did most of the work here herself, with a little guidance from us. The message is that if you are willing to put in the work of changing your lifestyle in significant ways, improved headache control (and improved health in general) is achievable with a minimum of medications.

Chapter 9

Migraine in Children and Adolescents

Migraine is not just an adult condition. Something like 5% of all children have migraine, which amounts to around 2 million children in the United States. As pointed out in Chapter 2, the ratio of girls to boys with migraine is about 1 to 1—very different from adulthood, when women are more than three times as likely to have migraine as men.

Distinctive Aspects of Childhood Migraine

The manifestations of migraine in children may differ from those in adults. For one thing, the headache may not be as prominent as the nausea, and the actual headaches may be shorter— as brief as 2 hours, which is unusually short for adults. Several scientists have begun to see links between migraine in childhood and conditions such as abdominal pain, recurrent bouts of nausea, and even colic. If these links are real, this is welcome news for parents of children with colic and abdominal problems, since known treatments for migraine might well be effective against them. Unfortunately, the anti-nausea medications that work in adults are more likely to cause side effects in children, such as motor restlessness (jitteriness) and dystonic reactions (uncomfortable muscle contractions, especially in the neck).

Younger children are less able than older ones to characterize the details of their headaches and may be able to articulate only how "bad" or "sick" they feel. They may not remember where their headache pain was, when the last headache occurred, or what seemed to trigger it. Hence it is even more important for parents of children with migraine than for adult migraineurs to keep an accurate headache diary. The important information to share with the medical team includes (1) on which days the child had headaches, (2) how severe the headaches got, (3) how long the headaches lasted, (4) what other symptoms (like stomach upset) were happening, and (5) what triggers might have been present.

Adolescents are of course much more able to express their symptoms and how they affect their activities. But with the many physical, psychological, and social events happening in their lives, they may show even more frustration when headache control is not good than younger children do. The following case may sound familiar to parents of teenage migraine sufferers:

> Riley is a 15-year-old freshman at a highly ranked high school, where she is a straight-A student, plays on the girls' junior varsity field hockey team, is a student government representative, and is active in several after-school clubs. She began having severe headaches with nausea last year, and they now occur 3 or 4 times per month, many around her menstrual periods, which are fairly heavy. She treats her menstrual cramps with acetaminophen, which she says "is of zero help with my headaches!" She is quite frustrated and highly critical of her parents, who recently divorced. She stays up very late to "get all my work done" (which includes updating her Facebook page, preparing documents for student council, writing poetry, and doing homework), drinks several cups of coffee daily, and eats a poor diet. She sleeps late on weekends to "catch up." Her headaches

bring on nausea and sometimes vomiting, and her parents (between whom she splits her time) complain that during her headaches she becomes very irritable and is "mean" to her younger brother. She has recently become a strict vegan and refuses even to take medication that may contain animal products.

Clearly, Riley is an impressive girl who was taking the world by storm until her migraines started up. She needs help figuring out what might constitute triggers for her headaches, what lifestyle changes might reduce the problem, and what her options are for stopping a headache in its tracks. She is facing a number of challenges outside of migraines—her parents' divorce, painful menstrual periods, and all the usual slings and arrows of high school life. While most teens are reluctant to engage in psychotherapy, a good family therapist could be of enormous help here.

Prevention and Treatment

Box 9.1 summarizes key lifestyle strategies for children and teens with migraine. Children, especially teens like Riley, benefit from regular sleep schedules. Making wake-up time consistent is a good way to begin to enforce good sleep habits. Wake-up time can slide a little on weekends but should not be more than an hour later than on weekdays. Some teens have real problems falling asleep, and melatonin, a naturally occurring sleep aid, can be useful in the 1- to 5-mg range at bedtime. They should minimize their use of caffeine, which not only alters sleep cycles but can actually worsen migraine if the intake is either high (more than one cup daily) or varies. Electronic games and

> **BOX 9.1** Lifestyle Strategies for Preventing and Controlling Migraine in Children and Adolescents
>
> Regular sleep cycles, especially with regard to wake-up time; limited caffeine
>
> Regular mealtimes: no snacking or skipping meals
>
> Regular exercise: 3 days per week minimum, for 30 minutes each day
>
> Avoiding becoming overheated
>
> Good hydration, with electrolyte drinks to replace sweating loss if necessary
>
> Plans for emotional support during times of stress

emotionally charged videos might best be curtailed several hours before bedtime.

Regular meals are also essential for migraineurs, so dieting can be a real problem if it includes skipping meals. This is doubly true for any kind of eating disorder involving purging, which might be unknown to parents. Vegetarian diets are praiseworthy, as they usually represent adolescents' urges to live an ethical, healthy life; however, they can stimulate migraine if not done carefully. Vitamin supplements, especially B12, are important, and it is a good idea to involve the family physician in the design of the diet.

Exercise seems to be really helpful in combatting migraine. Riley is probably doing better with headaches than she would if she were sedentary. Paradoxically, however, excessive exercise can bring on headaches. What we usually tell our patients is that if they want to do vigorous exercise, they should build up to it—what trainers call conditioning. Here is a story about a frustrated young man who is finding a direct link between exercise and his headaches:

> Clay is a 17-year-old starting midfielder for his high school's soccer team; he is also the team captain. He finds that during practices (which take place four or five times a week after school) he begins to develop a migraine headache, which becomes severe by evening. The new coach has ramped up the training regimen, and Clay thinks that might be the problem. However, he feels that as captain he has to set an example and push himself as hard as everyone else during practice. He never gets headaches after games or even after light runs. His headaches tend to improve somewhat with ibuprofen, but they make it hard for him to study in the evening.

Here the heavy training regimen seems like the culprit, and it could be very beneficial for Clay's parents to visit the soccer practice and see how extreme it gets. An interesting approach might be for Clay to try indomethacin prior to heavy exertion. This medication is something like the ibuprofen he already takes (so it would be something of a substitute), but it has been found to prevent exercise-induced migraines in many people. Of course he will need to use it sparingly and under a physician's guidance, but it could spell the difference between success and failure as team captain.

Medication options for relieving and preventing migraines in children and teens are similar to those used for adults (see Chapters 5 and 7), including beta blockers, antidepressants, and anti-seizure medications, although evidence that these work in children is limited and some evidence suggests that certain preventive drugs for adults may be ineffective in children. One very safe medication that seems to effectively prevent migraine in children is cyproheptadine (Periactin). The triptans are probably safe for adolescents and even for children, but most have not been studied as well in those groups as in adults, so consulting with a physician about their use is generally best. Rizatriptan is approved for children over 6 years old, and almotriptan is approved for adolescents. There is good evidence that sumatriptan nasal spray is safe in adolescents as well.

Managing the Impact of Childhood Migraine

As with adults, chronic pain in children can wreak havoc not just on the pain sufferer but on the family and other social systems surrounding the individual. Parents can feel helpless and depressed, and friction often arises when they differ regarding the best medical and non-medical approaches. The situation can be even harder with parents not living together, and of course in those cases there may be two sets of adults in the parent role. Siblings can feel sympathy and anger at the same time, since the family tends to focus on the "sick" child to the exclusion of other family members. Even grandparents and extended family can be highly affected, as the child's migraines can prevent or at least alter expected family events. The child or adolescent with migraine, keenly aware of the unfairness of it all and feeling sorry for her- or himself, also feels a burden of guilt over being the cause of time-consuming and costly medical care along with all of the other sacrifices made by the family. These are not easy conflicts to solve, and counseling can be invaluable, both individual and family based. Support groups for child and teenage migraine sufferers have cropped up as well, and these can be very helpful.

Children do best when they see that there are plans to try to keep their headaches to a low frequency and for what to do when headaches hit. Adolescents generally like to have more control over their condition, but they also need a structured program, especially one including their lifestyle. When simple measures such as those described in this chapter do not meet the needs of the child or adolescent migraineur, a visit to a headache center for further advice is generally very worthwhile.

Chapter 10

Migraine During Pregnancy
and When Breastfeeding

Because migraine is so common in women during childbearing years, migraine during pregnancy is an important "women's issue" deserving of its own chapter. When pregnant women use medications to treat acute headache attacks or to prevent headaches, there can be concerns about exposure of the fetus. Levels of risk vary among medications, and we prefer to be very conservative when making recommendations to women who are contemplating pregnancy. Having reasonable treatment plans in place prior to pregnancy is ideal, since about two-thirds of pregnancies are unplanned. Other issues specific to female patients are the use of contraception and using medications during breastfeeding.

Most migraineurs have migraine without aura, and the majority of pregnant patients of this kind see an improvement in their headache pattern, especially during the second and third trimesters. Presumably this improvement is due to the rise in stable, high levels of estrogen as the pregnancy progresses. Many of our patients are delighted to be pregnant, as they have learned to expect this improved headache pattern at least during the pregnancy. This is especially true for women who have menstrually related migraine, where menses is a trigger or headaches only occur around menses.

Other patients, however, experience worsening or new migraine symptoms or have concerns about medication use during and after pregnancy. Let's look at some illustrative cases.

Anna, recently married, was doing quite well with her headaches until she developed some daily nausea and morning vomiting. She missed her period and wondered if she might be pregnant. Her doctor confirmed the positive results of a home pregnancy test, and Anna and her husband were delighted by the news. However, she is concerned about potential harm to the baby because she used several doses of sumatriptan (Imitrex) just before she realized she might be pregnant. She raises this concern during a visit to her headache doctor.

Our next patient is suffering from a dramatic exacerbation of one of her migraine symptoms.

Linda is about 7 weeks pregnant. Her migraines seem to be slightly less frequent than before her pregnancy, but when she gets an attack she has a lot of vomiting. During a particularly long attack, she has vomited so much that her husband has brought her to the emergency room. The couple are uncertain what to do and hope the emergency room physician can help.

A third patient is experiencing new pain symptoms.

Kayla has migraine attacks with aura. Before or during some of her headaches she sees an enlarging blind spot (basically a dark hole) with a shimmering edge in her vision, which lasts for about 30 minutes. She is in her second trimester of pregnancy, and her headache frequency has not improved.

The attacks, some of which last 2 days, are occurring 3–4 times a week. Vomiting does not relieve her headaches. She has had so many attacks that, she reports, her head and neck feel "sore"; it even hurts to put her head on the pillow. Her nurse-midwife has sent her to the headache clinic in hopes of getting her some safe relief.

As we will relate at the end of the chapter, all of these women got effective treatment for their headache attacks and had pregnancies with good outcomes.

Three Phases of Migraine Management Surrounding Pregnancy

Before Pregnancy

Some pregnant migraineurs still have problematic headaches, and these need to be dealt with. Ideally, we try to get non-pharmacologic measures in place even before pregnancy (see Chapter 8). These often require the involvement of a psychologist, who might help the patient with techniques such as biofeedback (hand warming or muscle relaxation), relaxation exercises, or cognitive behavioral therapy. These techniques are best tailored to the particular patient: not all patients benefit from the same technique. They may be used either without medications or with selected medications; they are not "anti-pharmacologic" but can be complementary to medications (the two approaches may work synergistically).

During Pregnancy

Frequent headaches with disability and especially vomiting can be a serious issue during pregnancy, as well as afterward during lactation and breastfeeding. If treatment is necessary the patient and her healthcare providers need to work together to choose an appropriate option, balancing benefits in controlling the headache versus risks to the fetus. Ob-gyn doctors and pediatricians use many resources to assess these relative benefits and risks. We will discuss some of these resources later in the chapter.

After Delivery

The time just after delivery can be a rocky time for women with migraines. Schedule changes, changing hormone levels, lack of sleep, and stress can all trigger migraine. Additionally, there are concerns about using medications during breastfeeding, as all medications get into breast milk. Making a plan in advance and adjusting it depending on how matters unfold is the best way to manage the challenging time just after the baby's birth.

Medication Use and Risks

Although as a rule of thumb we prefer all our pregnant patients to have learned non-pharmacologic techniques to help manage their headaches (as discussed above and in Chapter 8), sometimes these techniques are not sufficient by themselves to relieve or prevent migraine, and certain drugs and procedures may be necessary to get control of the attacks. We try to use the fewest and the safest medications possible, balancing the risks (to the fetus and to the mother) against the benefits. Vomiting leading to dehydration is a risk to the pregnancy and should be controlled, with medication if necessary. We prefer for the patient to be able to manage her attacks herself, but other measures can be taken if a trip to the doctor's office or emergency room becomes necessary.

BOX 10.1 Traditional FDA Categories of Medication Risk in Pregnancy

A: No risk, as shown by controlled human studies

B: No evidence of risk in humans, but no controlled studies

C: Risk to humans not ruled out

D: Positive evidence of risk to humans from human or animal studies

X: Contraindicated in pregnancy

The FDA has for many years categorized medications according to the risk they pose during pregnancy. Originally letter categories (A, B, C, D, and X) were used (see Box 10.1), but in 2015 the Pregnancy and Lactation Labeling Rule replaced these with three subsections, which hopefully provide better practical information for pregnant patients and their healthcare providers (see fda.gov/downloads/Drugs/GuidanceComplianceRegulatoryInformation/Guidances/UCM425398.pdf). This approach is still being phased in, especially for newer drugs, so many clinicians also refer to the older categories. Drugs in categories B and C are often used during pregnancy if the benefit outweighs the risks. Drugs in category X should be avoided, as "the risk of use in pregnant women clearly outweighs any possible benefit of the drug," according to the FDA. Drugs in category D are often avoided as well, although "the potential benefit of the drug in pregnant women may be acceptable despite its potential risks."

Clinicians may use other resources as well for information about medication risks during pregnancy and during lactation

---

BOX 10.2 Commonly Used Migraine Medications Listed by Type of Risk Associated with Use in Pregnancy

Category A: none

Category B: acetaminophen, cyproheptadine, metoclopramide, ondansetron, lidocaine (for nerve blocks)

Category C: triptans, promethazine, amitriptyline, butalbital, prochlorperazine, gabapentin, zonisamide, propranolol, tizanidine, onabotulinumtoxinA

Category D: valproate, divalproex, topiramate

Category X: ergotamine, dihydroergotamine

---

and breastfeeding, such as Teris (depts.washington.edu/terisdb/) and LactMed (toxnet.nlm.nih.gov/newtoxnet/lactmed. htm). Pregnant women and women of childbearing ability are often excluded from drug trials, so relevant information about many drugs is limited or even nonexistent.

Box 10.2 lists the safety ratings for common migraine medications. For treating most headache attacks during pregnancy we recommend acetaminophen (category B except when given intravenously) and promethazine (category C). Most patients are aware that these can be taken orally as pills, but many are unaware that they can also be used rectally, as suppositories, for attacks with severe nausea or even vomiting. These medications are reasonably safe and very effective. Because of the possibility of medication overuse headaches, we try to limit their use to 2–3 days per week.

Some physicians are now allowing the use of triptan drugs during pregnancy. There are data indicating that using sumatriptan (Imitrex) and zolmitriptan (Zomig) in particular may be reasonable in some patients. We are not yet fully convinced of this. However, data from the sumatriptan pregnancy registry (pregnancyregistry.gsk.com/sumatriptan.html) do suggest that there is no increased risk of poor fetal outcomes when this drug is inadvertently taken early during pregnancy.

Sometimes daily preventive medications need to be considered if headaches remain too severe, too frequent, or too disabling. One of the safest preventive medications during pregnancy is probably propranolol (Inderal). It is category C, as is the calcium channel blocker verapamil. Topiramate (Topamax) and amitriptyline (Elavil) have been downgraded to category D and so are best avoided during pregnancy if possible. The ergot drugs ergotamine (Cafergot) and dihydroergotamine (DHE-45) are category X and should be avoided in pregnancy: they decrease uterine blood flow to the fetus. Valproate (Depakote) is clearly teratogenic (i.e., it causes birth defects), and we generally avoid it even in our patients who might become pregnant. There are no preventive drugs in category A (completely safe during pregnancy), but one older drug, cyproheptadine (Periactin) is category B and often can be helpful in reducing headache frequency and improving sleep; however, it is not recommended during lactation.

In our headache clinics we employ a procedure called *occipital nerve blockade* with pregnant women to treat acute severe migraine attacks and also to reduce the number or severity of attacks. The occipital nerves can be found at the base of the skull and run up over the back of the head. They are often exquisitely tender during a migraine attack as well as at other times in some patients who suffer from frequent attacks. In occipital nerve blockade, an anesthetic (lidocaine) is injected around the nerves to produce temporary anesthesia locally. The procedure poses very little risk and sometimes can result in an improvement in the headache pattern for many weeks. Treatment can be repeated regularly if the benefit is significant. You can read more about nerve blocks in Chapter 12.

Sometimes, for refractory (treatment resistant) headaches, a short course of a steroid such as prednisone may be offered to break the persisting headache pattern. A single course carries little risk; however, we avoid repeated administration, which has serious potential side effects, including gastrointestinal bleeding. If there has been repetitive vomiting with dehydration, intravenous fluids may be administered. This is usually done in infusion suites or the emergency room, although we have occasionally admitted patients to the hospital for inpatient treatment for this problem.

The headache pattern may again change immediately after the baby has been delivered. Simple measures aimed at ensuring adequate rest and sleep, regular meals, and other non-pharmacologic approaches are obvious and fundamental strategies during this time.

Treating Migraines While Breastfeeding

All medications get into breast milk to some extent, and some pose a potential risk to the baby. The American Academy of Pediatrics has guidelines about medications that can be used during breastfeeding. The pumping/discarding ("pump and dump") method can allow many mothers take their medications just after breastfeeding to minimize exposure to the baby. Lactation consultants can be very helpful in designing plans. Ideally, recommendations regarding medication during breastfeeding should be overseen by the pediatrician. Most pediatricians feel that sumatriptan and zolmitriptan are safe as well as acetaminophen, ibuprofen, naproxen, propranolol, riboflavin,

---

BOX 10.3 Medications and Supplements Likely to Be Safe
for Breastfeeding

Acetaminophen
Ibuprofen, Naproxen, Diclofenac
Sumatriptan, Zolmitriptan, Eletriptan
Metoclopramide, Promethazine
Ondansetron
Lidocaine (for nerve blocks)
Magnesium
Riboflavin

---

and magnesium. Box 10.3 lists these and other medications likely to be compatible with breastfeeding.

Migraine in Pregnancy: Some Successful Examples

Let's go back to the three patients we discussed at the start of the chapter and see how their problems were dealt with.

Anna's ob-gyn told her that the sumatriptan pregnancy registry data show no increased risk of bad outcomes from exposure to sumatriptan during early pregnancy. This reassured Anna greatly, and by the end of the second month of her pregnancy her headaches ceased entirely. She delivered a healthy baby boy.

When Linda went to the emergency room she was dehydrated. After the emergency room physician gave her intravenous fluid as well as 1 gram of intravenous magnesium, her headache stopped. She was also given an injection of promethazine to stop her vomiting. Linda was sent home with promethazine and acetaminophen suppositories, and using these she found she could terminate all her subsequent migraine attacks at home. She had a healthy baby.

Kayla was rather miserable when she arrived at the headache clinic. The back of her head was sore, and she had been vomiting. The nurse practitioner performed a pair of occipital nerve blocks (one on each side of her head) and gave her an intramuscular injection of promethazine for her nausea. Her headache stopped immediately, and she was sent home with acetaminophen and promethazine suppositories. The benefit from the nerve blocks lasted for just over 3 weeks, so for the remainder of her pregnancy Kayla made visits to the headache clinic every 3–4 weeks or so, obtaining excellent control of her headaches from the nerve blocks. Like our other mothers, she delivered a healthy baby.

Chapter 11

Chronic Migraine

As discussed in Chapter 2, when we talk about migraine being "chronic," we are referring not to how long the patient has had headaches but rather to how often the headaches occur. The International Classification of Headache Disorders has a formal definition of chronic migraine which can be summarized as follows: For at least the past three months, 15 or more days of headaches per month, most of which have migraine features.

The criterion that at least half of the headaches must be migraine is debatable, since some of us feel that if you have migraine, *all* your headaches are migraine. Obviously, there are exceptions—for example, a person unlucky enough to develop a new neurological condition may develop a truly new headache type, which can be an important clue that medical evaluation is warranted. (See Box 11.1 for a list of techniques that can be used in evaluating people with frequent migraines.) One of our colleagues from Canada likes to say, "Migraine hijacks your nervous system"—meaning that if a migraineur gets a headache while ill, the headache will likely fit into the patient's migraine pattern.

Chronic migraine has received a lot of attention among headache experts, in part because it seems in many ways to be much worse than episodic migraine (migraine occurring on fewer than 15 days per month). Much research and many resources are now being devoted to trying to understand how chronic migraine differs from episodic migraine. So let's think

BOX 11.1 Evaluation of Chronic Migraine

History and examination (general, neurologic)

Imaging: usually brain MRI, perhaps MRI of neck

Lumbar puncture ("spinal tap") for measurement of spinal fluid pressure and tests for infection or inflammation

Blood tests sometimes useful: thyroid tests, erythrocyte sedimentation rate (test for inflammation), tests of kidney function (blood urea nitrogen [BUN], creatinine), tests of liver function (liver enzyme levels), complete blood count, Lyme test.

about some "facts" about migraine and how frequency may affect how these conditions affect migraineurs. First, however, let us once again consider some examples to illustrate what we'll be discussing.

Tom has had migraines since the first grade (he always remembered how embarrassing it was to vomit in front of his classmates then). They occurred 3–4 times per month until he went to medical school, when they increased in frequency to 10–12 times per month. After his mentor at the medical school put him on amitriptyline, his frequency improved to about 8 times a month until he entered residency training, when sleep deprivation and stress pushed his headache frequency to about 20 days per month. It seems the amitriptyline no longer helps.

Our next patient's headaches, unlike Tom's, have been chronic from the start.

Marcia's migraines have occurred more than half the month since their onset during college. She saw several doctors, who prescribed a variety of ineffective preventive regimens, including propranolol (Inderal), which made her depressed; amitriptyline (Elavil), which made her "fat"; verapamil (Calan), which made her constipated; and valproate (Depakote), which made her gain even more weight and gave her a tremor, both of which resolved after discontinuing it. She also had acupuncture (which helped for 6 weeks only) and saw a chiropractor, a "reflexologist," and several massage therapists. Nothing seemed to work. She has held several jobs but was absent from work so often she lost them all. Now Marcia's fiancé has brought her, at age 34, to the headache clinic. He is concerned about their relationship, because she is ill most of the time. He is also "freaked out" because she hurts all over—even her "hair hurts." He takes this last symptom as a sign of a psychiatric problem.

Marcia's headache diary, shown in Fig. 11.1, reveals just how frequent her headaches were.

Our final patient was especially desperate.

Carol arrives at our headache clinic from out of state on Christmas Eve. She is 47 years old and has traveled a great distance because of what seems to her a hopeless headache condition. She is the last patient of the day during a snowstorm, so she will be unable to get home for the holiday. She is a lifelong migraineur, but until the past couple of years her headaches were always infrequent, perhaps 4–5 per year (although when they did occur, they were severe). After her fiancé died in an accident years ago, she never married; she now is "alone in the world" save for her cat, Fluffy. She found fulfillment through her work at the local hospital, most recently

Sunday	Monday	Tuesday	Wednesday	Thursday	Friday	Saturday
[ ]	[ ]	[1]	[2]	[3] 5 N	[4] 7 N, S	[5] 3 N
[6]	[7] 6 N,S	[8] 6 N, S	[9]	[10] 10 S, P	[11] 4 N	[12] 3
[13] 4	[14]	[15] 7 N, S	[16]	[17] 4 N	[18]	[19] 7 N, S
[20] 8 N, S	[21]	[22] 7 N, S	[23]	[24] 7 N, S	[25] 9 N, S, P	[26]
[27]	[28]	[29] 5 N	[30] 4→8 N, S	[ ] 6 N, S	[ ]	[ ]

FIG. 11.1 Headache diary of a chronic migraine patient, showing headaches on most days. Pain level is rated on a 1–10 scale, with level 10 defined as the most severe pain possible. (Note the variation in severity of headaches.) N, S, and P refer to medications used by this patient to attain relief of headache, nausea, or both (N = naproxen, S = sumatriptan, P = promethazine).

as a medical coder. Two years ago she developed lung cancer, which was treated by surgery, chemotherapy, and radiation and is now in remission. During her treatment for the cancer, her migraines increased "with a vengeance"; they are now daily. She is so disabled by them that her employer reluctantly had to fire her for absenteeism. This has been devastating for her, as her only friendships were with her coworkers. She feels isolated, has become depressed, and confides that were it not for Fluffy, she would just as soon end it all.

How Chronic Migraine Develops

It seems that "migraine begets migraine"; in other words, if the frequency is increasing unchecked, it tends to keep increasing. Some experts distinguish between episodic migraine (occurring 9 or fewer days per month) and "high-frequency episodic migraine" (10–14 days per month); it is high-frequency episodic migraine that tends to become chronic migraine. This increased frequency of migraine is sometimes called "chronification." Less than 5% of episodic migraine patients progress into the chronic migraine category each year, but as the number of patients with chronic migraine seems to be stable, one can assume that about as many chronic migraineurs revert back to the lower, episodic frequency.

In the United States somewhere between 3 million and 9 million people have chronic migraine (some of whom have other forms of chronic daily headache, such as chronic tension-type headache). It is two to three times more common in women than in men. Chronic migraine is a major public health concern: Compared with individuals with episodic migraine, chronic migraineurs have more disability and a lower quality of life, develop more psychiatric problems, and use more healthcare resources. As a result, not surprisingly, they have more absenteeism and more "presenteeism" (being at work but performing at lowered effectiveness) in the workforce than their co-workers without migraine. Chronic migraine also negatively affects family and other personal relationships.

Who is at risk for converting from episodic to chronic migraine? Among the most likely are patients with an increasing frequency of headaches, patients who overuse acute symptomatic medications (see Chapter 5), and patients with what is called *allodynia*—when something that does not normally hurt becomes painful (such as wearing your glasses or earrings, putting your head on the pillow, even your hair). Allodynia may result when pain pathways in the brain are overactive. Migraineurs with high-frequency episodic migraine and allodynia are especially likely to convert to chronic migraine. Other risk factors are obesity (and the more you weigh, the worse the risk); thyroid disorders (whether hyper- or hypothyroidism); snoring and sleep

---

BOX 11.2 Risk Factors for Migraine "Chronification"

Obesity (risk increases as weight increases)

Childhood maltreatment

Family history of migraine

Low socioeconomic status

Snoring and sleep apnea

Being unmarried

Being a woman

Excessive caffeine intake (more than 2 cups a day)

Medication overuse

Stressful life events: work changes, moving, change in marital status or relationship, family strife

Psychiatric conditions: uncontrolled PTSD, anxiety, depression, bipolar disorder

History of head injury

History of neck injury

Thyroid disease

---

apnea; excessive caffeine use (more than 100 mg daily); head trauma; and psychological stressors (such as change in marital status; problems in the family, especially with children; moving; and changes or problems at work). Box 11.2 lists these and other risk factors for developing chronic migraine.

Treatment and Management

Ultimately, we consider chronic migraine more disabling and harder to treat than episodic migraine. Patients with chronic migraine are often angry, frustrated, and desperate (and so are their healthcare providers). They often come to our clinics after having many negative tests and failing many treatments. Sometimes they resort to unproven therapies. As mentioned above, families are harmed as well by the impact on the migraineur. This certainly sounds like a hopeless situation.

The good news is that it is *not* hopeless. An "evidence-based" approach to the problem often leads to improvement. This usually requires finding an interested and knowledgeable healthcare team to work with you and your family. The approach must be comprehensive. In our clinics we address all the issues listed in Box 11.1. We start with a thorough history and examination and usually obtain MRI images of the head, and often the neck as well. We stop overuse of medications. Sometimes we admit the patient to the hospital for several days to give intravenous medications to stop the headache. A lumbar puncture (spinal tap) may be performed to ensure that the spinal pressure is neither high nor low. (We have seen many cases of abnormal spinal fluid pressure that were missed for years but, once diagnosed, permitted steps to be taken that resolved the headaches.) The point is to be thorough and, frankly, aggressive enough to get control of the situation.

Sometimes we use our colleagues in the pain clinic to treat neck and other pain. Surgery on the neck simply for pain is rarely helpful and often may even worsen the pain. (Surgery may, however, be indicated if there are deficits on the examination such as arm or leg weakness or loss of control of the bowel or bladder.) Instead, our pain clinic colleagues can often improve neck pain without surgery by performing various procedures directed at pain pathways.

Confounding psychiatric issues are also evaluated and treated. Anxiety, depression, bipolar disorder, and phobias occur with increased frequency in migraineurs. Diagnosing and treating these problems are often crucial in improving a migraineur's overall situation. We check for sleep disturbances and treat them if found. Sleep disturbances are abundantly common in migraineurs, including trouble falling asleep; trouble staying asleep; nightmares in those who have post-traumatic stress disorder (PTSD); restless legs syndrome; and sleep apnea (especially in those who are obese). Improving sleep almost always seems to improve the headache pattern.

Part of dealing with chronic migraine involves the use of preventive therapies. The best evidence in the medical literature suggests that the two treatments most likely to be effective in this situation are topiramate (Topamax) and injection of onabotulinumtoxinA (Botox). Therefore we generally start with one of these. Other preventive treatments discussed elsewhere in this book might work but are less likely to, based on the evidence.

Topiramate is an anticonvulsive (anti-seizure) medication that was initially used to treat epilepsy but was later found to be useful in preventing migraine (both episodic and chronic). Unlike most other preventive agents, it is not associated with weight gain and therefore is a popular choice, especially if patients are overweight. In fact, many patients lose weight on this drug, which is useful. The target dose is approximately 100–200 mg daily, far less than usually used for epilepsy. Occasionally it causes significant "mental fog," which may include word-finding problems, confusion, or forgetfulness. If this occurs, one should reduce the dose or consider stopping the drug. More frequently, topiramate causes tingling in the hands and feet, for which a possible antidote is potassium (so eating bananas, tomatoes, or even molasses can help). Topiramate can cause kidney stones to form in some who are predisposed. Very rarely it can cause an attack of acute glaucoma, resulting in severe eye pain; this is a medical emergency and requires a trip to the emergency room.

As Botox, onabotulinumtoxinA is well known to the public, especially for its cosmetic uses. It is the only medication approved by the FDA for treating chronic migraine; therefore most medical insurance plans cover it in appropriate circumstances. Other forms of botulinum toxin do not have FDA approval for treating chronic migraine and have not been sufficiently studied to recommend them. The dose of Botox is specified at 155 units, and the injection strategy is standardized: it is administered at 31 locations in the forehead, sides of the head, back of the head, upper neck, and shoulders (Fig. 11.2). Botox takes just a few minutes to administer (about 6 minutes in our hands). The procedure is repeated every 3 months. The treatment is usually very well tolerated, and side effects are relatively uncommon; they include neck discomfort, droopy eyelid, double vision, an

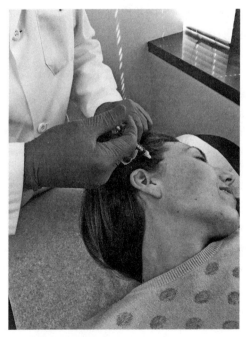

FIG. 11.2 A patient having a Botox injection.

elevated eyebrow ("Spock eyebrow"), and flu-like symptoms. If any of these occur, they go away in a few days or, less commonly, a few weeks. Long-term study of recipients of this treatment suggests that at 2 years most patients still receive benefit from the injections and continue using them, while about 10% stop using them for lack of continued benefit. A substantial minority (about 25%) do so well that they revert to an improved headache pattern (less than 15 days per month) and can discontinue the injections.

Chronic migraine is a serious medical condition, so it is important to tackle this disease head-on. When a comprehensive approach involving the patient and a knowledgeable healthcare team is taken, most patients benefit.

Successfully Managing Chronic Migraine: Some Examples

Let's revisit our cases from the start of the chapter and see how they turned out.

Tom is now a physician. The driver for the "chronification" of his migraines seems to have been sleep deprivation and stress. He saw his doctor, who ordered a thyroid test and an MRI because of Tom's worsening headaches; fortunately, the results were normal. Tom's amitriptyline dose was increased and Botox was added to his treatment. Over the course of 6 months, his headache frequency decreased from about 20 days per month to 6–7 days monthly, and he found he could control all his headaches with a triptan drug (sumatriptan). After a year, the Botox was successfully discontinued. Tom is meticulous about getting enough sleep to the extent he can.

Marcia's care was also successful. Her nurse practitioner obtained a brain MRI and thyroid tests, which returned normal results. After topiramate was chosen for prevention, Marcia's headaches improved and she lost 20 pounds. Her hair also stopped hurting. The nurse practitioner explained to Marcia's fiancé that this symptom is a form of allodynia related to having such frequent migraines. Marcia had reduced absenteeism and improved work performance; a year after starting topiramate, she actually got a promotion with a pay raise.

Carol's case had an especially moving resolution—we sometimes call it "A Christmas Carol" (with apologies to Charles Dickens). After taking a careful history, we learned that that during her cancer treatment, Percocet (acetaminophen plus oxycodone, a narcotic) had been begun for her postsurgical incisional pain. Coincident with daily use of the Percocet, her headaches increased to the point that they were now daily. Carol found that whenever she missed a dose, her headache got even worse, so she was still taking this drug, even though her surgery was 2 years ago and her incision was no longer painful. Her examination results from her primary doctor were normal, but the situation was desperate (and so were she and her doctors!). On her Christmas Eve visit, the doctor at the headache clinic stayed late and admitted her to the hospital. All tests there again returned normal results. Her Percocet was stopped, and she was treated with intravenous medications for 3 days. Back home, a friend of hers visited her house to feed her cat. By the second hospital day her migraine had stopped and she was feeling much better. She was discharged to her home and over the next few months had only 3–4 headaches per month, all of which she could control. The hospital where she had worked took her back, and she resumed the work she loved doing in the company of her friends.

Carol continued in this improved state for 3 years, until her cancer returned. Two weeks before she died, she sent the headache clinic a letter thanking her doctor for "restoring my dignity." She worked until several weeks before her death. Her doctor still sees patients on Christmas Eve.

Chronic migraine can be devastating. Fortunately, there is hope. Most patients can be helped; success depends on persistence, knowledge, and compassion.

Chapter 12

Newer and Experimental Treatments for Migraine and Other Headaches

Migraine is one of the most common medical problems in the world, and disability from migraine has been estimated to be similar to that from illnesses like stroke and heart disease. Despite this, research funding from government and other sources has been woefully inadequate. Gifted medical investigators in the public and private sectors have nonetheless been developing new ways to prevent and lessen the pain of migraine. In this chapter we will share information about new medications, new forms of and new delivery systems for older medications, and newer methods for preventive and acute treatment of migraine like nerve blocks and electrical and magnetic stimulation.

To prepare for our look at these advances, let's think about a case of a person who has "tried everything" and would really like to hear about new ideas being developed for treating migraine.

Sonjay is a 42-year-old software engineer who has been having migraine headaches since his early 20s. They used to occur once a month during college but have been much more frequent over the last 2 years. He thinks the increase might be due to high levels of stress at work: he was promoted to a management position, which brings a lot more responsibility and time at work along with the salary boost. He gets a severe throbbing headache with some nausea, dizziness, and "mental fog" at least 2 days per week, and some weeks he seems to have daily headaches. He has tried beta block-ers, antidepressants, other blood pressure medications, anti-seizure medications, many vitamin supplements, acu-puncture, chiropractic, Botox, and all of the triptans. Over-the-counter medications have no effect, and even when he goes to the emergency room for particularly severe head-aches, the medical staff there have trouble controlling his pain. The medication that seemed to help most was topi-ramate (Topamax), but it caused more mental fog; antide-pressants were also a bit helpful but made him too sleepy. He says he is "desperate" because his job is at risk from his headaches.

New Forms of Medication

There is actually a lot of hope for Sonjay. Already, a number of pharmaceutical companies are producing new forms of some medications that have been around for a while. What is the advantage of these new forms? First, many medications avail-able for acute treatment of migraine are in pill form and there-fore tough to use when nausea is present. Also, there is some thought that in some migraine sufferers, absorption of oral medication is impaired during their headaches by a phenom-enon called *gastroparesis* (which means "stomach paralysis"). Medication that bypasses the stomach and intestinal tract avoids these problems.

Injected medication does this but is cumbersome and may require the help of another person. Also, many people are very uncomfortable with injections. Nasal spray forms of medica-tion are a natural option. Two of the triptans, sumatriptan and zolmitriptan, have been available as nasal sprays but have only become popular in this form with a few migraineurs. A new device that uses a person's own breath to "push" sumatriptan into the nasal cavity may hold promise. Another clever alternative is an inhaled preparation of dihydroergotamine (DHE), a very potent anti-migraine agent previously available only in injectable form. The inhaler will look very familiar to asthmatics, who know how to inhale useful medication.

Another recently available product was a skin patch that used an electrical current to "push" medication through the skin into one's circulation—a process called *iontophoresis*. Unfortunately, this product caused skin burns in a small number of people and had to be removed from the market. Another new formulation of an older migraine remedy is a dissolving powder form of diclofenac. One empties a little packet into a small glass of water and drinks it. A number of our patients seem to prefer it over the traditional pill forms.

A very exciting new field in the medical treatment of a number of illnesses involves the injection of antibodies against abnormal or problematic substances in the body. These "monoclonal antibody" therapies have been used effectively in treating cancer, arthritis, and inflammatory bowel disease. The antibodies must be injected, because oral forms would simply be inactivated in the intestinal tract. Fortunately they are long-acting and need only be administered about once per month. In migraine, the body chemical being targeted for monoclonal antibody treatment is calcitonin gene–related peptide (CGRP), and initial results with this approach seem highly promising.

Nerve Blocks

Nerve blocks have been used for decades in the treatment of headaches. They are done via injection of a mild anesthetic agent, much like the procaine (Novocain) that dentists use when performing procedures. The anesthetics used for headaches are usually bupivacaine and lidocaine; sometimes a small amount of steroid medication is used in addition. It is not clear why putting scalp nerves to sleep (generally the occipital nerves, in the back of the head) would help relieve a migraine. Even more puzzling is why nerve blocks sometimes prevent future migraines long after the anesthetic effect has worn off. Nonetheless, most headache specialists have used nerve blocks for many years for patients with difficult to treat migraines. Generally nerve block procedures are done right in your physician's office and take not more than a few minutes (Fig. 12.1). Side effects are minimal, though some people may get a little woozy. Box 12.1 lists the nerves that can be anesthetized in nerve block for headache treatment.

A new device allows a small amount of a local anesthetic to be dripped onto the tissues in the back of the nose, where a number of important nerves are located. Fig. 12.2 shows a patient undergoing this painless procedure. Early results are very encouraging and show virtually no side effects of any concern.

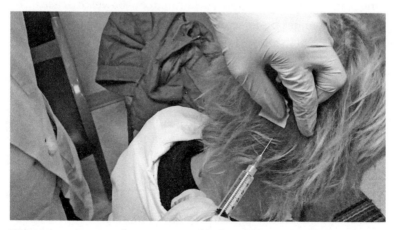

FIG. 12.1 A patient having a nerve block—in this case, of the occipital nerve.

BOX 12.1 Common Nerves Blocked by Headache
Specialists

Greater occipital nerve
Lesser occipital nerve
Auriculotemporal nerve
Supraorbital nerve
Supratrochlear nerve
Sphenopalatine ganglion

Nerve Stimulation

The success of nerve blocks in migraine patients has led a number of researchers and clinical specialists to think about using electricity to *stimulate* nerves. This concept may seem puzzling,

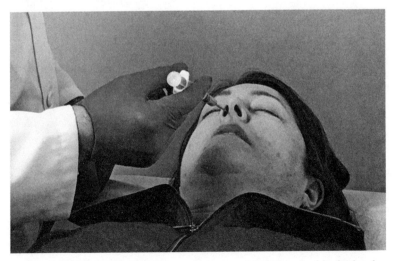

FIG. 12.2 A patient undergoing an intranasal infusion for blockade of the sphenopalatine ganglion.

since it would appear to be the opposite of anesthetizing nerves. And it is—except when one considers that in the brain and in peripheral nerves there are often conflicting activities, some of which may promote head pain and some of which may lessen it. Most of the nerves that have been targets of nerve blocks have also turned out to be good sites for stimulation.

Stimulation can be done as a trial using a temporary stimulator, and if it seems to help, a permanent stimulation system can be inserted. This usually consists of small metal electrodes surgically implanted near the nerve and connected to a generator placed somewhere in the upper back or chest. However, the electrodes can break, move to inactive sites, or become infected; also, the generator can fail or require battery replacement. There is very little evidence for the usefulness of these devices

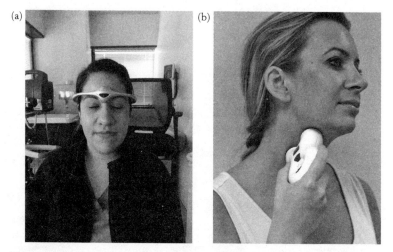

FIG. 12.3 Noninvasive electrical stimulation. (a) A migraine sufferer using the Cefaly. (b) Another migraineur using a handheld vagus nerve stimulator. (Photograph used by permission of Eric Liebler, electroCore.)

in headaches, but for patients who have not responded to any other form of treatment they offer real potential.

There is mounting interest in so-called noninvasive electrical nerve stimulation, which does not require implanted electrodes or batteries. One device, called the Cefaly (Fig. 12.3a), is worn like a headband and stimulates nerves in the forehead. Another, handheld device can be used to stimulate the vagus nerve in the neck at the time of headache (Fig. 12.3b). Evidence for the efficacy of these approaches is not yet firm, but both are worth watching.

Magnetic Stimulation

Magnetic stimulation of the brain has already shown promise in treating severe depression, and several centers have been experimenting with it for treating patients with difficult-to-control migraines. The procedure requires no implanted electrodes or generators, is painless, and seems to be without much in the way of side effects. The patient holds the stimulator device over the back of the head and presses a button to apply the magnetic field (Fig. 12.4). Researchers are considering use of this kind of device at the time of headache as well as regularly as a migraine prevention strategy.

Infusions and Hospital Treatment

Migraine sufferers who experience frequent headaches become frustrated very quickly if preventive and acute treatments are not helping. One option that some headache specialists can

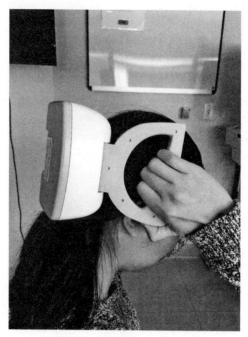

FIG. 12.4 A patient using the eNeura transcranial magnetic stimulation device.

offer is to administer intravenous medication aimed at ending the headache attack. Sodium valproate (Depacon) is one medication that can be given through an intravenous line in an outpatient infusion center. Generally this is done once daily for up to 3 days and may go a long way toward stopping some patients' daily headaches.

If infusion of medications like sodium valproate is not helpful enough, we sometimes bring patients into the hospital for several days to use even stronger medication to break headache cycles. Hospitalization can be remarkably helpful even when every other approach has been disappointing. Box 12.2 lists some of the medication options that can be used during hospital stays.

BOX 12.2 Medications Used During Hospital Treatment of Unremitting Migraine Headaches

Dihydroergotamine (DHE)
Chlorpromazine
Lidocaine
Ketamine
Divalproex
Magnesium
Dexamethasone

Progress and Patience

What we often tell our patients who are struggling with frequent disabling headaches, like Sonjay, is to be patient, as advances in migraine treatment do seem to be happening, albeit slowly. We understand this can be of small comfort. Nonetheless, some of the new ideas discussed in this chapter, especially nerve stimulation and antibody approaches, have the potential to revolutionize our field. Stay tuned.

Chapter 13

Tension-Type Headache

The "Usual" Headache

In Chapter 14 we will discuss unusual types of headache—some quite rare, others just less common than migraine. But first we thought we should describe what we might call the "usual headache": tension-type headache (TTH). This is the most common headache type. Migraine is the third most common disease in the world, but TTH is the second, affecting more than three-quarters of all people.

What Is Tension-Type Headache?

Box 13.1 shows some of the characteristics of TTH. This kind of headache can affect people relatively infrequently, anywhere from just shy of 15 days a month to a few times a year or less, in which case we call it "episodic," or it can be "chronic," occurring on 15 or more days per month, even daily or constantly. Despite being such a common condition, TTH is very poorly studied; compared with migraine, it is not at all well understood. The International Classification of Headache Disorders defines it essentially as the headache that is not migraine. It usually occurs on both sides of the head, does not throb, is usually mild to moderate in severity, and does not bring on nausea or vomiting. It is not made worse by exercising. While

---

BOX 13.1 Characteristics of Tension-Type Headache

- Known by many other names: e.g., tension headache, muscle contraction headache, stress headache
- Defined as headache that is not migraine
- "Episodic" if occurring less than 15 days per month; "chronic" if occurring 15 days or more per month
- Lasts minutes to days
- Often on both sides of the head and has a "pressure" quality, as if the head were in a vise
- Often mild to moderate in severity; non-disabling; sometimes improves with exercise
- May include sensitivity to light or sound, but not both; lacks most other migraine features, such as nausea or vomiting

---

not dramatically severe, these headaches are often quite persistent; when people talk about "nagging" headaches, they usually mean TTH.

Patients with infrequent TTH generally do not go to their doctors, as they are almost always able to treat their headaches themselves with simple remedies, including those bought over the counter (or "off the shelf"). However, people with chronic TTH do seek medical attention for their stubborn, difficult-to-treat headache pain. In this case, a thorough examination of the head and neck is performed, and sometimes blood work and head imaging as well.

Let's look at a case of TTH:

Judy is a 44-year-old office manager who has come to see us on the recommendation of her primary care physician.

Her first words to us are "I'm not sure why I am here. All those people in the waiting room look much sicker than me!" For the last 10–15 years she has been having daily or near daily headaches, which she thought were due to her stressful job: "I have four bosses, and they all want different things! By the end of the day, my headache has built up to a level where I just want to go and collapse." She has found that a glass of wine, some acetaminophen, or just relaxing are usually enough to help her get to the point of minimal pain, so that she can fall asleep. "But" she says, "this is getting old!" She adds, "I should own stock in Tylenol." She has no other real complaints and no indications for other causes of headaches. Results of her neurological exam are normal. Her head pain tends to extend from her forehead around to her temples on each side and to the back of her head.

Fig. 13.1 shows the diagram on which Judy indicated her "band-like" pain pattern. We'll return to Judy at the end of the chapter to see how things turned out for her.

Mimics of Tension-Type Headache

We often see TTH in patients with other kinds of headaches, which can make diagnosis and treatment challenging. Moreover, various kinds of headache can masquerade as TTH (Box 13.2). In diagnosing TTH one must especially take care to rule out three other headache types. Headache due to giant cell arteritis (GCA), also known as temporal arteritis, can start and look like any type of headache, including TTH. GCA occurs nearly exclusively in patients 50 years of age or older, and there is a blood test (erythrocyte sedimentation rate, or

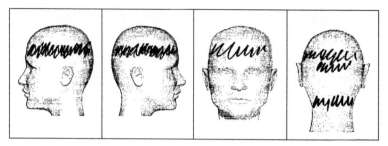

FIG. 13.1 Patient-drawn diagram of tension-type headache with "band-like" pain around the head.

ESR) to screen for it. It is important not to miss this condition, because half of the people with it will go blind if not treated promptly and effectively. A second situation that mimics TTH is analgesic rebound headache in migraineurs who are overusing some of their acute medications. Their headache pattern

---

BOX 13.2 Mimics of Tension-Type Headache

- New daily persistent headache (headache that just begins one day and lasts more than 3 months)
- Hemicrania continua (constant one-sided headache that responds to the medication indomethacin)
- Cervicogenic headache (headache due to problems in the neck)
- Post-traumatic headache (can resemble any type of headache)
- Headache due to mass lesions, giant cell arteritis, high or low cerebrospinal fluid pressure, temporomandibular joint disease, sleep apnea, hypothyroidism, or medication overuse (analgesic rebound)

will have changed from isolated episodes of migraine to a background of constant or near constant headache that looks like chronic TTH with superimposed attacks reminiscent of their migraines. Third, the vexing entity new daily persistent headache (NDPH, discussed further in Chapter 14) can look exactly like chronic TTH except for the way it starts abruptly, like switching on a light switch, one day and then is continuous from onset until it (sometimes) mercifully stops just as abruptly.

Treating Tension-Type Headache

Treatment of TTH has not been studied as well as migraine management has. Only one treatment has a good evidence base supporting its use in treating chronic TTH: the drug amitriptyline. It seems clear that adding relaxation training provides further benefit. Nortriptyline, a cousin of amitriptyline, has been helpful for many of our patients as well. Migraine treatments such as beta blockers and triptans have been very useful for many TTH patients, which of course brings up the possibility that some TTH sufferers have migraine as well or even that their headaches, while resembling TTH, are actually mild migraines in disguise. Other medications that seem to help some TTH sufferers are topiramate and venlafaxine

Since chronic TTH can lead to daily use of painkillers, it is important that patients not overuse potentially harmful medications such as non-steroidal anti-inflammatory drugs (NSAIDs) like aspirin and ibuprofen, which can cause gastrointestinal bleeding and kidney failure. Non-pharmacologic measures like biofeedback and exercise may be helpful instead.

Box 13.3 summarizes pharmacologic treatments for TTH.

> **BOX 13.3** Pharmacologic Treatments for Tension-Type Headache
>
> For episodic TTH: aspirin, acetaminophen, other NSAIDs (e.g., ibuprofen, naproxen sodium) at times of more severe pain
>
> For chronic TTH: amitriptyline, nortriptyline, topiramate, venlafaxine

Successfully Managing Tension-Type Headache: An Example

Let's see how the considerations above entered into the diagnosis and treatment of our patient Judy. She was not really old enough for GCA and did not have the "start date" phenomenon characteristic of NDPH. There was no family history or any other evidence for migraine, so we decided she was a relatively pure TTH sufferer. (We know of no French-sounding word like "migraineur" for that—perhaps "tension-neur"?) Clearly her headaches were reducing her quality of life: one thing we have learned is that daily headache, even if relatively mild, is maddening. We recommended a combination of amitriptyline taken at bedtime and instruction in mindfulness relaxation by a therapist. The combination of these interventions, along with a bit more assertiveness regarding her job duties at work, led to a dramatic reduction in Judy's headache frequency and, in her words, "lots more up-time," By the way, her "band-like" head pain is considered typical for TTH, but we have seen various patterns, including one-sided headaches and, perhaps most commonly, generalized pain over the entire head.

Tension-type headache, given its frequency and the significant disability it can cause, deserves medical attention. Hopefully, we will start to understand the mechanisms of this common medical problem as researchers study it a bit more.

Chapter 14

Unusual Headaches

Cluster Headache, Other Trigeminal Autonomic Cephalalgias, and New Daily Persistent Headache

In this chapter we are going to discuss some types of headache that can be very troublesome but are less common than migraine. There are over 300 different types of headache, some very "unusual." Here we are going to focus on the category of **trigeminal autonomic cephalalgias (TACs)** and the perplexing entity of **new daily persistent headache (NDPH)**. Both are considered "primary headaches," since they have no known cause. They are important, because they can be missed during diagnosis and generally require specific treatment.

Here are a couple of examples of what we will be talking about.

Jack is a 47-year-old man who has come to the office crying because he is desperate. He is having about 8 headache attacks per day. They begin with pain that Jack rates as having an intensity of 10 (out of 10), always around his left eye. During the attacks, which last between 30 and 60 minutes, his left eye waters, his nose runs, and he paces about. He sometimes gives himself a shot of sumatriptan (Imitrex), but his insurance allows him only 6 doses a month. If he uses a shot, the attack goes away in less than

5 minutes. Some attacks awaken him, so he now dreads falling asleep. He has found that drinking a beer can set off his headaches. Jack started having these attacks at the age of 34. They used to occur daily for up to 6 weeks at a time, but afterward he could go many months without any headache. For the past 3 years, however, the attacks are happening nearly every day. Many preventive medications have failed to help, and he has run out of his sumatriptan injections.

Our second case is striking for the circumstances of its onset.

Ben is a graduate student who came down with a flu-like illness while traveling overseas. When the illness subsided, he noticed he had a headache. This headache has now been present for 7 months. Most of the time it is mild, "dull," and nagging, involving his entire head. However, about twice a week and for no apparent reason, the headache escalates to a severe, one-sided, throbbing headache that makes him nauseated for several hours, causing him to lie down. No over-the-counter medications he has tried, and nothing his doctor has tried, seem to help at all. All testing (blood work and MRI of his brain) has returned normal results. Ben is "exhausted" by these headaches, which his doctor thinks are migraines.

Trigeminal Autonomic Cephalalgias: Cluster Headache and Its Relatives

The TACs tend to be unilateral and accompanied by "autonomic symptoms," including tearing, nasal congestion, nasal drainage, and eyelid swelling. Box 14.1 lists various kinds of TAC.

BOX 14.1 Trigeminal Autonomic Cephalalgias

- Cluster headache: severe, one-sided headaches lasting 1–3 hours and occurring in cycles; more common in men
- Paroxysmal hemicrania: severe but shorter and more frequent one-sided headaches than in cluster headache; generally responsive to indomethacin
- Short-lasting unilateral neuralgiform (SUN) headache: very brief, one-sided attacks occurring many times per day; generally unresponsive to medication
- Hemicrania continua: constant pain over one side of the head; responsive to indomethacin

---

Cluster Headache

The best-known TAC is the **cluster headache** (Box 14.2). It is less than a hundredth as common as migraine: in a city of 100,000 people, there would be more than 10,000 with migraine but only about 70 with cluster headache. While uncommon, it is *very* important. The pain of cluster headache is said to be the worst pain known. Women who have had cluster headache have stated that the pain of childbirth pales in comparison—and unlike childbirth, cluster pain can occur multiple times a day.

Cluster headaches can be divided into two forms. In "episodic cluster," attacks occur essentially daily for several weeks or months, followed by weeks, months, or even years without attacks; these two phases are referred to as "bouts" and "remissions," respectively. In "chronic cluster," the patient has no attacks for a total of less than a month out of the year. In either form of cluster headache, individual attacks often occur

---

BOX 14.2 Cluster Headache

- Attacks of extremely severe pain on one side of the head, usually in or around the eye, lasting 1–3 hours
- Up to 8 attacks per day
- Often associated with restlessness or agitation (pacing, running)
- Other symptoms on the same side as the headache during attacks, possibly including red or watery eye, stuffy or runny nose, droopy eyelid, decreased pupil size, sweating or flushing of the face (or both), and full sensation in the ear

---

at particular times of day and sometimes awaken the patient at night. Also, the onset of bouts in episodic cluster often occurs near the longest and shortest days of the year and around when we change the clock for daylight saving time and back. In a given person, bouts tend to begin and to end at about the same times each year. Cluster headache has some relationship, then, to our internal timing mechanisms. This makes sense, because it looks likes the mechanism for cluster headache has something to do with problems in the hypothalamus, which is in some ways the brain's "biological clock."

The pain of cluster headache reaches its very severe maximum intensity either immediately after or very shortly after it begins. Attacks last 1–3 hours, and the pain is usually felt in or near the eye. Patients say they may feel burning, even a sensation like a "hot poker," in the eye. They may have a red eye, watery eye, droopy eyelid, stuffy nose, or runny nose and may be, among other things, extremely agitated, running about, screaming, or even banging their heads against the ground. The attacks may awaken them from sleep and therefore cause a fear of falling asleep. During bouts, alcohol and nitroglycerin may trigger attacks. It used to be reported that cluster headache was six to seven times more common in men than in women, but more recent reports suggest that the ratio is about 3 to 1, at least currently. Why this type of headache is more common in men remains unknown.

Cluster headache sufferers can feel hopeless and even suicidal. However, there are effective treatments. We get brain MRIs on every cluster patient, because occasionally they reveal causative abnormalities, often around the region of the pituitary gland. When such causative lesions are found, we say the headaches are "symptomatic." Treating the underlying cause may cure the headache.

Every patient with cluster headache deserves a healthcare provider who is expert in managing this terrible disorder. There are also patient resources specifically for cluster headache sufferers (see Chapter 17).

Relieving Acute Cluster Headache

Several treatments can quickly shut down acute attacks of cluster headache. Those that work fastest are obviously best. Subcutaneous injections of sumatriptan (Imitrex) work very fast, and the 4-mg dose can be used up to 3 times a day (if the patient does not have coronary artery disease or angina). This treatment is unfortunately very expensive, and often the cost prohibits patients from receiving help—a good example of medical system failure, in our opinion.

Delivering 100% oxygen by mask (not nasal prongs or cannula) also works but sometimes requires very high flow rates (up to 20 liters per minute). This antidote also can be expensive, and often medical insurance will balk at paying for it (Medicare does not cover it at this time). One danger with oxygen inhalation is that oxygen is flammable, and many cluster patients are smokers. They must therefore remember to not smoke anywhere near the oxygen apparatus. (We had one patient admitted to a hospital burn unit for smoking *while* using oxygen!)

Oral narcotics work only minimally in cluster headache and should be avoided whenever possible, because they can cause serious problems with addiction.

Many patients entering a cluster bout benefit from so-called bridge therapy. Sometimes occipital nerve blocks are helpful (see Chapter 12). A short course of oral steroids such as prednisone for a week or so may also reduce the attacks or, if the patient is lucky, terminate the bout. If these simpler options are ineffective and the patient is having many attacks, a brief admission to the hospital for intravenous medication (usually dihydroergotamine [DHE] given repetitively over several days) can be helpful.

Preventing Cluster Headache

Preventive drugs are often employed to reduce the frequency, severity, and duration of cluster attacks. The most effective is verapamil, a calcium channel blocker that is otherwise often used to treat high blood pressure. Sometimes higher-than-usual doses of verapamil may be necessary to get effective relief. Many other medications can be used alone or added to verapamil, but the evidence for their efficacy is weak. These medications include lithium, valproate (Depakote), topiramate (Topamax), and lamotrigine (Lamictal). Sometimes a large dose of melatonin (up to 10 mg) at bedtime helps suppress nighttime attacks.

When desperate patients suffering from acute cluster headache are admitted to the hospital for intravenous medications, as discussed above, preventive drugs can be started simultaneously. Prolonged benefit, even for weeks after the admission, is sometimes achieved.

Surgery and Devices for Treating Cluster Headache

Nerve stimulation (Chapter 12) is beginning to be studied for use in cluster headache as well as migraine. In the most invasive options, electrodes are implanted under the skin near the occipital (and sometimes other) nerves and connected by wires to an implanted electrical "pulse generator." The stimulation can reduce or turn off the cluster headache in some patients. Data supporting use of such occipital nerve stimulation techniques are limited, and they are considered experimental by insurance companies. These procedures are quite expensive, and as we mentioned in Chapter 12, there can be problems such as infection and breaking or migration of the wires, leading to failure of the stimulators.

Stimulators of the vagus nerve and sphenopalatine ganglion are also being tested for cluster headache. They are potentially safer and more reliable options, as they do not require nearly as much instrumentation.

For truly refractory patients another option, with more risks, is **deep brain stimulation**, pioneered in Milan, Italy, by Dr. Massimo Leone and his colleagues. A small number of the most severely affected cluster patients have had electrodes implanted deep in their brains (near the hypothalamus). Electrical stimulation via these electrodes has helped some of these patients. The technique has significant risks, however, such as infection, bleeding, and even death.

Paroxysmal Hemicrania

Another TAC condition is *paroxysmal hemicrania* (Box 14.3). This type of headache seems like cluster headache at first, but attacks are a little briefer (2–30 minutes) than in cluster headache and occur a few more times a day. Some of the same features as in cluster headache may be present, such as tearing from the eye, nasal congestion, runny nose, and swelling around the eye. Paroxysmal hemicrania is often misdiagnosed as cluster headache, so if someone who is thought to have cluster headache does not respond to the usual cluster treatments, indomethacin (Indocin) may be tried. Indomethacin usually does not work in cluster headaches, but it works extremely well in paroxysmal hemicrania. Indomethacin is the most anti-inflammatory of the nonsteroidal anti-inflammatory drugs (NSAIDs), which include ibuprofen and naproxen sodium. It can be very hard on the gastrointestinal tract, causing heartburn

---

BOX 14.3 Paroxysmal Hemicrania

- Similar to cluster headache except that attacks are slightly briefer (30 minutes or less) and occur slightly more often per day
- Other symptoms on the same side as the headache during attacks, possibly including red or watery eye, stuffy or runny nose, droopy eyelid, decreased pupil size, sweating or flushing of the face (or both), and full sensation in the ear.
- Dramatic therapeutic response to treatment with indomethacin

and even gastrointestinal bleeding. The lowest effective dose is therefore used, and measures to protect the stomach are usually also employed.

Like cluster headache, paroxysmal hemicrania may be episodic, with bouts and remissions, or chronic, with a relatively unremitting pattern (with periods of freedom from headache lasting less than a month).

Short-Lasting Unilateral Neuralgiform Headache

A type of TAC producing brief but sometimes extremely frequent attacks is **short-lasting unilateral neuralgiform (SUN) headache** (Box 14.4). The attacks are again one-sided, occur around the eye, and produce red or watery eye. Attacks are very brief (1–600 seconds) but can occur even more frequently than in paroxysmal hemicrania—up to dozens per day. SUN headaches are

---

BOX 14.4 Short-Lasting Unilateral Neuralgiform
Headache

- One-sided headache, usually in or near the eye, similar to cluster headache and paroxysmal hemicrania but briefer still, lasting from 1 second to 10 minutes; may be experienced as "stabs" or jolts
- Frequency of attacks varying from 1 per day to dozens per day
- Other symptoms on the same side as the headache may include red or watery eye, stuffy or runny nose, droopy eyelid, small pupil, sweating or flushing of the face (or both), and full sensation in the ear

---

very hard to treat; lamotrigine may be the most effective overall treatment, and sometimes intravenous lidocaine gives temporary relief.

Hemicrania Continua

Last in this group of TACs is the often misdiagnosed **hemicrania continua** (Box 14.5). This is another one-sided headache, but it is constant. At its least painful it is mild to moderate in severity, but it may worsen for minutes to hours to a severe headache that often seems like a migraine (pounding, with symptoms of nausea, vomiting, sensitivity to light, sensitivity to sound, or some combination thereof). With the worsening of the headache the sufferer's eye may water, the nose may become stuffed up or run, and other symptoms may occur, all

---

BOX 14.5 Hemicrania Continua

- Constant, one-sided headache that has lasted more than 3 months
- Generally very mild to moderate in severity, but with attacks of worsening (exacerbations) to moderate to severe pain, possibly with features of migraine
- Other symptoms on the same side as the headache during attacks, possibly including red or watery eye, stuffy or runny nose, droopy eyelid, decreased pupil size, sweating or flushing of the face (or both), full sensation in the ear
- May be associated with agitation
- Dramatic therapeutic response to treatment with indomethacin

---

on the same side as the headache. Hemicrania continua can sometimes have remissions (periods of time without daily headache).

Hemicrania continua can be misdiagnosed as cluster headache, migraine, or even both. Like paroxysmal hemicrania, hemicrania continua responds dramatically well to indomethacin (and usually not well to much else).

New Daily Persistent Headache

The last type of unusual headache that we will discuss is NDPH. This headache is often not diagnosed correctly, so its exact prevalence is uncertain. However, it is commonly seen in specialty headache clinics. In essence, this is a headache that begins one day and persists for at least 3 months (Box 14.6). It may look like tension-type headache or migraine or have features of both. Some patients relate having had some sort of infectious illness before the onset of the headache, but it not known if there is a relationship between the two occurrences. The cause of NDPH is unknown, and it usually does not respond to medical treatments.

BOX 14.6 New Daily Persistent Headache

- Begins one day and persists for more than 3 months; may look like tension-type headache, migraine, or both
- May follow an event such as a viral infection or surgery
- Often does not respond well to any treatment
- Sometimes spontaneously remits (stops on its own), although it may recur later

---

Results from routine testing, including blood tests, MRI, and analysis of spinal fluid, are usually normal. In many patients the pain suddenly ceases after months to years of constant headache. Occasionally, in some unlucky patients, it returns.

Treating Unusual Headaches: A Success and a Failure

Let us see what headache types our two cases from the start of the chapter had and what was done to try to help them.

Jack, who described having numerous very severe headaches lasting 30–60 minutes each every day for 3 years, had chronic cluster headache. All preventive treatment tried had failed, and he could not get enough sumatriptan injections to control his numerous attacks. In situations like this, some cluster patients become suicidal. His nurse practitioner and his doctor decided to admit him urgently to the hospital. His sumatriptan was stopped, and his acute attacks were treated with high-flow 100% oxygen by mask. He was treated with intravenous DHE 3 times a day, and within one day his attacks stopped. Because DHE is an ergot drug, his doctor discharged Jack on another drug of this type, oral methylergonovine (Methergine). After discharge, his medication was adjusted over several days, and at a follow-up appointment 2 weeks after discharge his headaches were found to be mostly controlled.

Ben, sadly, had NDPH. His doctor did a thorough evaluation and could find no underlying cause. Multiple medications were tried, but none were helpful. He saw two other headache specialists, but no one could defeat these headaches. Most of the time he could pursue his studies, but occasionally he would have to go home from the office and rest for the remainder of the day. About 16 months after his headaches began, they diminished over several days and then one day just stopped; they have not returned. This is not that unusual for NDPH. We wish headaches of this type spontaneously disappeared more often, since patients with them are so difficult to help.

As you have seen, some of the unusual primary headaches we discussed in this chapter have very effective treatments, while others, like SUN headaches and NDPH, do not respond well to any treatment. To ensure that you receive appropriate care for your headache condition, it is crucially important that someone do a thorough evaluation and make the correct diagnosis. In Chapter 16 we will discuss how to find an effective medical team and communicate with its members for the best chance of success in dealing with your headaches.

Chapter 15

Head Injuries and Headache

There are nearly 2 million emergency room visits in the United States every year for head injury. Most of the injuries are what we call "minor" or "mild," meaning that there was no fracture of the skull, bleeding inside the brain, or any other serious consequence, like prolonged coma. However, even mild head injuries can result in ongoing headache problems.

Concussion

Eric is a 29-year-old, recently married young man who recently moved into a new house with his wife. He was working in his garage 2 months ago and, while moving some boxes, struck his head on the partly closed garage door. He stumbled and felt dazed but did not lose consciousness. He was "out of it" for the rest of the day, and the next morning he continued to feel mildly confused and was having a new headache, which he experienced all over his head. He therefore went to the emergency room, where he was evaluated and otherwise found to be in good health. A CT scan of his head showed normal results. He was given acetaminophen (Tylenol) for pain. His confusion disappeared in a couple of days, but his headaches have persisted on a nearly daily basis since his injury. He has tried a number of over-the-counter medications and has seen several doctors, who have not been able to help him. He reports that his sleep has been "choppy"; sometimes he wakes up in the middle of the night with headache. Even though he continues to work in his job as a restaurant manager, he sometimes forgets to complete important tasks there and loses his temper even over "little things"—behavior that was not typical for him before the head injury.

Eric had a **concussion**, which is best described as *a mild head injury followed by either a loss of consciousness or any change in consciousness, such as being dazed or "seeing stars."* Concussions can cause any number of long-term consequences other than headaches, but in fact, headaches are the most common residual effect. These can affect part of the head or the entire head and can be frequent or infrequent. The headaches themselves are often nondescript, but they can resemble migraines and even include migraine features such as nausea, vertigo, and other neurological problems.

Treatment of these "post-concussive" headaches is challenging, but if they have some migraine features most headache specialists tend to treat them as if they were migraine. Beta blockers (like propranolol), cyclic antidepressants (like amitriptyline), and antiepileptic medications (like topiramate) have all been effective for some patients. Unfortunately, a large number of people with post-traumatic headaches prove to be very resistant to most medications; these people can become intensely frustrated. That may be why Eric became irritable.

Other interventions that can provide a great deal of relief for post-concussive headaches include occipital nerve blocks (see Chapter 12), manual approaches such as massage, and meditative techniques (see Chapter 8). Eric in fact benefitted enormously from some hard work learning muscle relaxation through the use of biofeedback, along with judicious use of pain relievers. Over the next 6 months after his initial visit in our headache center he slowly began to notice a reduction in his headaches to the point where he would experience a significant headache only around once a month. He noticed that his performance at work got better, and his wife confirmed that his mood improved so that he was now "his old self."

The Post-concussive Syndrome

The consequences of head injury, even when mild, can go far beyond the headaches that Eric experienced. Here is another, quite poignant story.

Matt is a 24-year-old army veteran who enlisted right after high school and was deployed to Afghanistan. While he was on active duty there, the vehicle he was riding in was hit by a grenade, and in the explosion he was thrown approximately 30 feet, landing on his back. When he was examined at a field hospital he was found to be a generally intact. A CT scan of his brain did not show damage. His cuts and bruises healed pretty quickly. Sadly, another soldier in his vehicle was killed in the explosion, and yet another lost a limb as a result of his injuries. Matt has experienced a number of symptoms since the explosion, including headaches, which he feels all over his head and are essentially constant. Even more problematic for Matt are his other symptoms, which include confusion, which comes and goes; difficulty concentrating; difficulty with reading comprehension; memory loss; and some fairly significant depression. He also has difficulty with sleep—both falling asleep and maintaining sleep throughout the night. Matt tried to return to his unit but was unable to regain his usual high level of functioning. Eventually he was sent home and discharged from the army because of his difficulties. He now carries a diagnosis of post-traumatic stress disorder (PTSD) and has been seeing a counselor. He is working stocking shelves at a local electronics store, but he finds it hard to even stay focused on this work and has had several poor reviews. His headaches are noticeable every day. He says he sometimes seems "withdrawn" to his coworkers and does not really "like socializing" with anyone other than his fellow veterans.

Matt seems to be suffering from post-traumatic headaches, but he certainly has many of the elements of a different, larger problem called the **post-concussive syndrome (PCS)**. This somewhat mysterious neurological condition is caused by mild or more severe head injury and can be quite devastating. Symptoms of the PCS tend to include headaches, memory and concentration difficulty, sleep problems, and mood issues (see Box 15.1). The current impression of why these problems occur has to do with the idea that the head injury included a transfer of force to the brain, leading to long-lasting or even permanent brain damage—so-called traumatic brain injury (TBI). The brain seems to have much less potential for healing from

---

BOX 15.1 Symptoms of Traumatic Brain Injury in the Post-concussion Syndrome

Headaches
Memory loss
Difficulty learning
Difficulty concentrating
Irritability
Depression
Sleep problems

damage like this than most organs do. Luckily, people with TBI may improve as spared parts of the brain gradually "pick up the slack." But this is a slow and sometimes incomplete process, and many folks who have suffered TBI are never quite the same. The PCS is beginning to be widely reported on in the media; you have almost certainly heard discussions about how to reduce it in student and professional athletes.

Unfortunately the PCS is quite difficult to treat. Certainly any headaches need to be reduced, and some reasonable approaches are outlined above and in previous chapters. It can be very difficult, however, to help with the cognitive challenges, which is understandable if there has been brain damage. One frustrating aspect of the PCS is that such damage is rarely seen on an MRI or CT scan. A few tests do illuminate some of the brain changes seen after TBI, such as positron emission tomography (PET) and the relatively new diffusion tensor imaging (DTI). Unfortunately, both of these techniques are expensive, and both are still difficult to interpret accurately in TBI.

BOX 15.2 Some Symptoms of Post-traumatic Stress Disorder

Recurring memories, dreams, or both of the traumatic event

Feeling distress in situations that remind one of the traumatic event

Avoiding situations that remind one of the traumatic event

Nightmares and insomnia

Depression, anxiety, feelings of guilt

Loneliness, detachment

Irritability, hostility, agitation, hypervigilance

In addition to PCS, Matt has PTSD. In fact, head injury with TBI is often accompanied by PTSD, because of the emotional toll the events surrounding the injury take on people. But in Matt's case, PTSD does not really seem to be prominent: he does not have the kinds of flashbacks, nightmares, and emotional difficulties that victims of emotional trauma often seem to have (see Box 15.2 for a list of typical PTSD symptoms). On the other hand, there are clues in his story to some possible social and emotional consequences of the events he lived through. Urging him to participate in "reintegration" or other counseling he would accept was wise.

The results of TBI can be devastating, including significant headaches that can be very challenging to control. Some of the symptoms can be "invisible" to others, including sleep and cognitive problems. On top of this, some of the symptoms we have seen in our patients with post-traumatic headache overlap with PTSD symptoms. So it is extremely important for victims of head injury to be evaluated by skilled neurologists and psychiatrists to make sure all important issues are identified and addressed.

Chapter 16

How to Communicate
with Your Medical Team

Achieving success in dealing with headaches is a very personal issue. Often headaches are not cured; rather, it is usually a matter of "managing" your headaches. Most patients want to deal with their headaches effectively and to be able to do much of that management by themselves. Therefore it is important for you as the patient to decide what you are seeking and then to try to find someone to cooperate with you in meeting your goals.

Sometimes a single healthcare provider may be all you need. Other times, especially if you go to a clinic, you may have a team of providers and their associates to deal with. In either case, there are some considerations to keep in mind before you "sign up" for whatever program you eventually choose.

Every team has a leader, whether it is a team of one (a solo provider, perhaps your family doctor or a neurologist) or a headache clinic (perhaps located at an academic medical center or university). There is even now a medical subspecialty called headache medicine, with credentialed physicians (certified by the United Council for Neurologic Subspecialties). The team leader must be knowledgeable, have sufficient resources to help you (access to testing and staff to help you obtain services and medications), and most importantly be interested in helping you manage your headaches—some physicians do not like seeing headache patients. If your primary care provider does not feel qualified to help you manage your headaches, is not interested in helping you, or is not having success in helping you, the provider may well refer you to another provider with whom he or she has had good experiences and who has had previous success in helping patients deal with headache conditions.

The Initial Visit

At your first doctor's visit related to your headache condition, you should expect an evaluation—generally a physical examination, including examination of the head and neck, and a neurologic examination. Your medical history should be obtained by an interview and should include any other healthcare providers you have previously seen or are currently seeing for this problem, results of any previous tests, and what treatments you have tried. Specifics are important. It is important to bring all your records as well as office notes, test results, and any images that have been made (such as CT scans or MRIs). (Box 16.1 outlines what to bring to your first visit.) Once the examination is performed, the history is taken, and results are reviewed, a diagnosis will be made. In other words, the key question "What type

---

BOX 16.1 What to Bring to Your First Headache Appointment

Headache calendar or diary for the past 3 months
Lists of previous medications tried (how much, how long)
Test results (including any MRI or CT scans on a disc)
Names of previous treating providers
Dates of hospitalizations and emergency room visits

of headache do I have?" will be answered—or at least a plan for answering it will be formed.

Assuming the doctor has arrived at a diagnosis, the next step is to set goals for managing your headache. This process is crucially important. You and your provider need to assess what treatment(s) to consider and then decide what you wish to accomplish. For any given treatment, headaches may improve (become fewer, milder, or shorter) but that improvement may come at some price (side effects). You and your provider should agree on what to expect and what to do if things do not go well. Any additional testing, medications, other treatments, or consultations are then ordered, and a follow-up visit is scheduled. Ideally, you will leave your first visit knowing who in the office to contact (and how) if you cannot get your medications because of insurance or cost issues, if you need to know a test result, if you have a side effect, or if you need to report any other problems (or successes!). If you aren't provided with a written treatment plan listing what medications to use and when to use them, what tests were ordered, and who to call if there are any problems, don't hesitate to ask for one.

Let's have a look at a couple of first-time visits with a headache specialist. The first example did not go well.

Emily is a thin, pale 41-year-old woman. Sitting stiffly, she states, "I am here because my doctor made me come." When asked about her headaches, she says, "I thought you already had my records." Not only is Emily unprepared to give a useful history of her headaches, but when asked specific questions she does not give detailed answers. A call to her primary care provider, who referred her, reveals that Emily was sent to the office because the primary doctor had discontinued prescribing narcotics for her headaches and that she is only in the office because she thinks she might get them during this consultation. When told that this is unlikely, she becomes tearful and storms out of the office.

Our second example offers a noticeable contrast with Emily's visit.

Todd is an overweight 52-year-old. He tells the headache specialist: "I am really glad to be here. My headaches have really been pretty awful over the past 6 months. I really need you to help me figure out how I can turn things around." He has brought his medical records and has written out a summary of key events that he thinks might help. He also has brought a log of his headaches for the last month. "My primary doctor wants to be in the loop," he says. "Can you send him a copy of today's visit note?"

These two very different stories had two very different outcomes. Emily was not interested in forming a relationship with a headache specialist. Her agenda was to get a particular prescription (which we felt was not likely to help her). Failing that, she simply chose not to participate. Todd, on the other hand, was enthusiastic and prepared to form a therapeutic partnership. He was organized and helped the headache specialist begin a treatment plan and a cooperative effort to manage his headaches.

What to Do Between Visits

It is important to maintain headache calendars or diaries to monitor your progress. This is your homework! It keeps everyone up to date as to whether you are getting better or not. A famous headache expert, now retired, would not see patients who came back to his office without their headache calendars.

How would he otherwise know for certain exactly how they were doing? Most of us are not so strict, but knowing the details is extremely helpful. Over the years we have had patients use paper calendars noting when their headaches were occurring, what the severity of the headaches was, and how long they lasted. More recently, smartphone apps have become available that may help people more reliably remember to fill out their calendars.

If you have a problem between scheduled visits, call the office and be precise in describing the problem. If you are having a side effect from a medication, for example, saying "I feel sick" is not particularly helpful. If you say something like "I am overly sleepy from this medication," your provider may know immediately how to help you (e.g., lowering the dose or replacing the medication with another, less sedating option). If you feel you must stop a medication, it is very important to let your provider know, so that other arrangements can be considered and no time is lost in helping your headaches.

The Follow-Up Visit

At follow-up visits you should have your headache calendars, which your provider should review (Fig. 16.1)—not doing so should cause you some concern! Based on how you are doing, adjustments might be made in the treatment plan. Follow-up is truly a time for cooperation: you and your provider should be on the same page, and if not, the goals for managing your headache should be revisited and perhaps changed. Please be sure to inquire about the results of any tests you have had. It is not OK to just assume the results were normal; sometimes things are overlooked, forgotten, or missed. Box 16.2 summarizes what to bring to a follow-up visit.

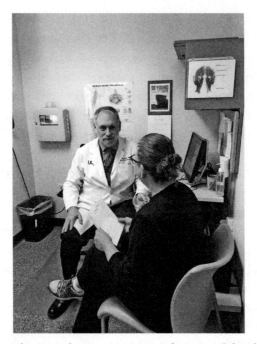

FIG. 16.1 A doctor and patient reviewing the patient's headache diary—a key part of follow-up.

Let's look at another patient's initial visit and first follow-up visit. As you'll see, things started out a bit tense with her but in the end were very productive.

BOX 16.2 Materials for Follow-Up Visits

Headache calendar or diary

List of medications you are currently taking, with dosages

Results of use of acute headache therapies (both good results and bad results or side effects)

Graziella is a 32-year-old mother of three, who was seen last month for the first time for her frequent headaches. At that visit she insisted on bringing her children in with her, who distracted her frequently. She argued that she needed to continue taking 4 tablets of Fioricet daily because "That is the only thing that helps me!" She was diagnosed with chronic migraine complicated by medication overuse. Her headache specialist explained medication overuse headache to her, went over some lifestyle strategies, and started her on a low-dose preventive medication. She forgot to take her headache diary with her when she left the office, and she had to call several times after this first visit asking for further explanations. At the first follow-up visit, Graziella reports that she continues to have frequent headaches, although fewer, and is down to 1–2 Fioricet tablets daily. She is not very happy with the situation, however, and says: "I can't go on! You've got to do something about my headaches!"

Her doctor inquired as to what resources Graziella could draw upon to help with her workload and stresses, and it turned out her mother and mother-in-law both lived nearby. During subsequent office visits, they took care of the children, allowing her to take better advantage of the information provided during the visits. At the second follow-up visit, she was doing better but did not really have adequate improvement, so a brief hospital admission was arranged to get her off the offending medications in a safe and comfortable way. After 5 months she was back to an episodic migraine pattern of 3–4 attacks per month, which she could control with either naproxen sodium (Aleve) or sumatriptan pills. Getting to this point took a great deal of hard work and patience on Graziella's part and careful listening and planning on the part of the medical team.

If You Have Problems with the Medical Team

Most of the time your interaction with your medical team goes well and you can expect improvement. Sometimes, however, things do not go well. Perhaps there is poor "chemistry" between you and the provider, or the office does not have sufficient personnel to help you between visits if there is a problem. Maybe the provider is unsure of your diagnosis or has tried a few things without good results. All of these scenarios can lead to frustration and bad feelings. If you have held up your end of the bargain in good faith, it is reasonable in such circumstances to request a second opinion or a referral to another provider. We routinely offer to arrange second opinions if patients are not having the desired result; in fact, we belong to networks of headache specialists we count on to help us help patients with complicated or refractory headache conditions.

What we have tried to suggest in this chapter is that there are optimal ways to approach your treatment team to promote the best possible outcomes for your care. To read more about this topic, go to headachejournal.org/view/0/toolboxes.html and find the excellent article "Your Visit to the Doctor: Achieving a Satisfactory Result," by Dr. John Rothrock. Lastly, Box 16.3 lists options for finding a headache specialist.

BOX 16.3 How to Find a Headache Specialist

Academic or university medical centers
Members of the American Headache Society
Listings of specialists in headache medicine certified by
the United Council for Neurologic Subspecialties

Chapter 17

Migraine Resources

In this, our final chapter, we wanted to share some information about resources available for people with migraine. These same resources can help people with many other types of headache. They are also highly useful for families and friends of people with migraine and other headache conditions. There are a great many resources that people with headaches can access, but some are better choices than others. We will try to direct you to information from more reputable organizations, realizing that we will inevitably omit some resources and emphasize others.

Prior to the advent of the Internet, many people relied on their healthcare providers and on books and other library resources for information on their medical conditions. While this is still largely true today, accessing the Internet opens up a whole new range of possibilities. However, just because you find something on the World Wide Web does not mean it is true; the good, the bad, and the ugly all can be found online. We advise caution but will try to direct you to some unbiased and reliable resources. Should you not be computer savvy, we suggest you visit your local public library. Most libraries now offer computer resources, and the librarians can help you find links to the websites we suggest.

For the purposes of this chapter we are not recommending commercial websites. Some headache sites are sponsored by pharmaceutical companies, and while some of these sites include very good features, not all of them are unbiased, and one of their agendas may be to direct you to a particular product or treatment the company sells. You certainly are at liberty to visit these websites for particular information; however, the sites we will suggest are educational and charitable, with no agenda other than to offer information in a balanced, unbiased fashion.

We start with the American Migraine Foundation website at americanmigrainefoundation.org, which is sponsored by the American Headache Society (AHS; americanheadachesociety.org). This nicely designed site is an excellent place to start finding information about migraine as well as other headache disorders. It includes educational articles on various headache conditions and links to other resources, including the patient support group the American Headache and Migraine Association (AHMA; ahma.memberclicks.net). The AHMA has meetings in various locations (often in conjunction with gatherings of the AHS), allowing you to network with other headache sufferers in person. It also has an online social media presence, so you can network with others via the Internet if you are so inclined.

The journal of the AHS, *Headache: The Journal of Head and Face Pain*, publishes a list of headache "toolboxes," which are patient-friendly information sheets on topics related to types of headache, headache treatments, and headache resources. These articles are free at the journal's website (headachejournal.org). The content is very useful, and healthcare providers often read these articles themselves and hand them out for patients to read. One of them, from February 2009, was written by one of this book's authors (M. L.) and lists headache websites. Included are descriptions of the sites for the British Association for the Study of Headache (BASH) and a British patient-support group, the Migraine Action Association. (The latter is a wonderful organization, whose newsletter is full of practical information and news about research on understanding and treating headache.)

Websites of other organizations, including the National Headache Foundation (headaches.org), the Headache Cooperative of New England (hacoop.org), the Headache Cooperative of the Pacific (www.hcop.com), the Organisation for Understanding Cluster Headache (OUCH; ouchuk.org), and the International Headache Society (ihs-headache.org) have some very useful information in their public areas.

The website of the United Council for Neurologic Subspecialties (www.ucns.org) lists headache centers around the country as well as board-certified headache medicine specialists. You can find these listings at the subpages dealing with headache medicine from the council's homepage.

If you access other sites and find information that you might act on, it is a good idea to let your healthcare provider know. Information from certain websites is incorrect, or at least misleading or biased, and it is best to be cautious. You should keep your healthcare provider aware of any concerns you may have about information you have found, but you should also just share with your provider any information you find interesting. Properly accessed, the Internet is a tremendous resource for people with headaches.

We sincerely hope not only that the information in this chapter is useful but that you have found that this entire book meets your needs in trying to better understand and obtain effective treatment for your migraines. Our goal, of course, is to make things better for you, for other migraine sufferers, and for all your families. If you liked our approach, please let us know by writing to us at our offices, and if you have suggestions for improving this book we would also very much appreciate them. Thanks.

ACKNOWLEDGMENTS

Creating a resource for patients like this one involves a number of tasks that must all have be coordinated. We also had to balance all of these tasks with our busy practice and teaching schedules. We could not have succeeded without the tireless support of our editors at Oxford University Press, Craig Panner and Emily Samulski. Thanks, Craig, especially for the overall advice on producing a book for patients—a very different project from the medical texts and research publications we have worked on in the past. And thanks to both of you for the many insightful comments on specific details of this book. Without them, this book would have been a much weaker work. We are very grateful for the guidance.

Thanks also to the production team at OUP for helping with the format and overall "look" of the book. We really had no idea what format and design would serve the reader best and are very happy with the ideas you put forth.

Thanks as well to the index compiler. Indexes are tricky things, and we wanted to give the reader a way to navigate this book without reading it cover to cover. We think you have succeeded in that goal.

We want to thank our wives and families for their constant support throughout our training and practice.

We want to gratefully acknowledge the teaching we have received from our mentors, the encouragement and support of our colleagues, and the dedication of our nurses and administrative staff, who have made it possible for our headache centers to flourish.

We want to thank our many students over the years—the medical students, neurology residents, and headache medicine fellows. You have helped us by reflecting and challenging our ideas and practices, and as a result we have grown enormously. This is also true for our thousands of patients over the many years we have spent in headache medicine. You have taught us much of what we know about managing headache disorders by way of your trust in our plans and your feedback about them.

ABOUT THE AUTHORS

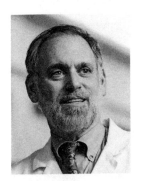

Dr. Morris Levin is a graduate of Stanford University, the Chicago Medical School, and the Albert Einstein School of Medicine Neurology Residency Program. He is a Professor in the Department of Neurology of the University of California, San Francisco (UCSF) and is the Director of the UCSF Headache Center. He is board certified in Neurology, with additional qualification in Pain Medicine (ABPN), and is board certified in Headache Medicine (UCNS) as well. He directed the Dartmouth Headache Center along with his co-author, Dr. Tom Ward, from 1998 to 2014 and was the Dartmouth Neurology Residency Program Director from 2000 to 2014.

He has written a number of medical journal articles and text-book chapters in the areas of headache and pain and is the author of *Neurology Clinical Case Studies* (Anadem, 2003), *Comprehensive Review of Headache Medicine* (Oxford University Press, 2008), and *Emergency Neurology* (Oxford University Press, 2013). He is the co-author of *Head, Neck and Facial Pain* (Anadem, 2006), *Educational Review Manual in Neurology* (Castle Connolly, 2006), *Headache and Facial Pain* (Oxford University Press, 2009), and *Refractory Migraine* (Oxford University Press, 2010).

Dr. Levin's particular clinical and research interests include headache diagnosis and classification, emergency neurology, traumatic brain injury, and medical education in neurology.

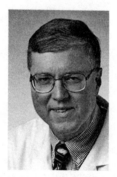

Dr. Thomas N. Ward grew up in Portsmouth, New Hampshire, where he attended the public schools. He subsequently graduated cum laude from Dartmouth College and with honors from Dartmouth Medical School. Dr. Ward trained at Albany Medical Center in internal medicine and then at Dartmouth Hitchcock Medical Center, where he did his neurology residency. He was later invited to establish and then direct the Dartmouth Headache Clinic. He was subsequently joined at that clinic by Dr. Morris Levin, who co-directed it with him for many years.

Dr. Ward is a Fellow of the American Headache Society and serves as the Editor-in-Chief of its journal *Headache: The Journal of Head and Face Pain.* He is also a Fellow of the American Academy of Neurology and of the American Neurological Association. Dr. Ward is a member of the Board of Directors of the Headache Cooperative of New England and serves as its Treasurer. He is currently Professor of Neurology Emeritus at the Geisel School of Medicine at Dartmouth. He resides in Norwich, Vermont, with his wife, Karen, and their Yorkshire terrier.

INDEX

References to figures, tables and boxes are denoted by an italicized *f*, *t* and *b*.

abdominal migraine, 30
acetaminophen, 4, 5, 56, 57
  acetaminophen/aspirin/
    caffeine, 74
  breastfeeding and, 110
  case stories, 92, 96
  isometheptene/
    dichoralphenazone/
    acetaminophen, 56*b*
  menstrual cramps with, 96
  oxycodone and, 123
  pregnancy and, 108, 108*b*, 112
  tension-type headaches,
    5, 140*b*
acupuncture, 67, 68*f*, 115, 126
adolescents. *See* children and
  adolescents
alcohol, 28, 28*b*, 87, 93, 147
Alice in Wonderland
  syndrome, 38
allodynia, 117, 123
almotriptan, 58*b*, 100

alternative treatment. *See* non-
  medicinal treatment
American Academy of
  Neurology, 72–73
American Academy of
  Pediatrics, 110
American Headache and
  Migraine Association
  (AHMA), 172
American Headache Society
  (AHS), 72, 172
American Migraine
  Foundation, 172
amitriptyline
  chronic migraine, 114–15, 122
  migraine preventive, 74, 76*b*
  post-concussive headache, 158
  risk for use in pregnancy,
    108*b*, 109
  side effects, 78*b*
  tension-type headache, 139,
    140, 140*b*

analgesic rebound headache, 14. *See also* medication overuse headache
angiotensin-converting enzyme (ACE) inhibitors, 79
angiotensin receptor blockers (ARBs), 79
antidepressants, migraine preventives, 76*b*, 77–78
anti-seizure medication, migraine preventives, 76*b*, 78–79
anxiety, 17
  antidepressants, 77–78
  chronic migraine, 118*b*, 119
  migraine patients, 28*b*, 31, 63, 72*t*
  post-traumatic stress disorder, 161*b*
aphasia, migraine aura symptom, 39*b*, 40
aromatherapy, non-medical treatment, 69
arteriovenous malformation (AVM), 11
  mimicking migraine, 26*b*
  MRI image of, 11*f*
aspirin, 15
  migraine attacks, 56
  non-medicinal types like, 69, 86
  tension-type headaches, 5, 139, 140*b*
asthma, 31, 72*t*, 73, 77, 81, 90, 127
atenolol, 76*b*
aura
  migraine phenomena, 37–41
  migraine symptoms, 39*b*
  phase of migraine, 27*f*, 29

bath salts, 16
behavioral medicine techniques, 70
benign intracranial hypertension, headaches, 12
Benson, Herbert, 89–90
beta blockers
  children and teens, 99
  migraine preventives, 76*b*, 77, 78*b*
  post-concussive headache, 158
  treatment, 89, 126, 139
biofeedback, 70, 90–91, 93
  hand-warming, 90
  patient practicing, 91*f*
  pregnant migraineur, 105
  tension-type headaches, 139
bipolar disorder, 72*t*
  chronic migraine, 119
  risk for chronic migraines, 118*b*
birch, 86
birth control pills, 79
blood pressure, 6, 73, 77, 126
  cluster headaches, 148
  headaches by, 9*b*, 17
  migraine preventives, 72*t*, 76*b*, 79–80
  stress and, 90
blood tests, chronic migraine, 114*b*
blood vessels, headaches and, 10–11
Botox. *See* onabotulinumtoxinA
brain malformations, headaches, 12
brain tumors
  headaches, 13, 25
  mimicking migraine, 26*b*

breastfeeding
  medications and, 103,
    106, 108
  treating migraines while,
    xvi, 110–11
British Association for the Study
  of Headache (BASH), 172
butalbital, 56*b*, 57, 108*b*
butterbur, 85

CADASIL (cerebral autosomal
  dominant arteriopathy with
  subcortical infarcts and
  dementia), 41*b*
caffeine, 56, 74
  children's use of, 97
  chronic migraine, 118, 118*b*
  non-medical treatment, 67–68
cajuput oil, 69
calcitonin gene-related peptide
  (CGRP), 127
calcium channel blockers
  case story, 83–84
  migraine preventive, 79–80
  risk for use in pregnancy, 109
camphor, 69, 85
candesartan
  benefits and undesired
    effects, 72*t*
  migraine preventive, 76*b*, 79
Cefaly, noninvasive electrical
  nerve stimulation, 130*f*, 131
cephalalgiaphobia, 62
cerebral autosomal dominant
  arteriopathy with
  subcortical infarcts and
  dementia (CADASIL), 41*b*
cervicogenic headache, 17, 138*b*
chamomile, 85–86
Chiari malformation, 12

children and adolescents
  aspects of childhood
    migraine, 95–97
  lifestyle strategies, 98*b*
  managing impact of childhood
    migraine, 100–101
  prevention and
    treatment, 97–100
chiropractic treatment,
    migraine, 87, 115, 126
chlorpromazine, hospital
    treatment, 133*b*
chocolate, 22, 27, 33
chronic migraine, 31, 113–14
  case stories, 114–16, 122–24
  definition of, 113
  development of, 116–18
  evaluation of, 114*b*
  headache diary of, 116*f*
  preventives, 80
  risk factors, 117–18, 118*b*
  treatment and
    management, 118–22
chronic tension-type headache,
    135, 136*b*, 139, 140*b*
chronification, migraines, 117,
    118*b*, 122
clonidine, 76*b*
cluster headaches, 2, 145*b*
  chronic, 145
  deep brain stimulation, 149
  description of, 146*b*
  episodic, 145
  nerve stimulation, 149
  preventing, 148–49
  primary headaches, 4*b*, 6–7
  relieving acute, 147–48
  surgery, 149
  trigeminal autonomic
    cephalalgia (TAC), 145–49

coenzyme Q10 (CoQ10), 89
combination medicines, 15, 44,
    56*b*, 56–57, 66, 74, 82
communication with medical
    team, 163–64
  case stories, 165–66, 168–69
  dealing with problems, 170
  doctor and patient, 168*f*
  finding a headache
    specialist, 170*b*
  first headache
    appointment, 164*b*
  follow-up visit, 167–69, 168*b*
  initial visit, 164–66
  what to do between
    visits, 166–67
computerized tomography
    (CT), 2, 3*f*, 13, 21, 157, 159,
    161, 164
concussion, 157–59
cortical spreading depression,
    37, 38*f*
cough headaches, 7
counseling, 100, 160, 162
CT scan. *See* computerized
    tomography (CT)
cyclic vomiting, 30
cyproheptadine
  for children, 100
  migraine preventives, 76*b*, 80
  risk for use in pregnancy,
    108*b*, 109
  side effects, 78*b*

deep brain stimulation, cluster
    headache, 149
depression, 31, 77
  antidepressants, 77–78
  chronic migraine, 119

  risk for chronic
    migraines, 118*b*
dexamethasone, hospital
    treatment, 133*b*
diazepam, rescue plan, 60*b*
diclofenac, 111*b*, 127
diclofenac potassium, 56
diet, 87, 92–93, 96, 98
dietary supplements, 89
diffusion tensor imaging
    (DTI), 161
dihydroergotamine
    (DHE-45), 57, 59
  case story, 82
  hospital treatment, 133*b*, 148
  inhaled preparation of, 127
  risk for use in pregnancy, 108*b*
  unusual headaches, 154
disability, related to
    migraine, 45–47
divalproex
  hospital treatment, 133*b*
  risk for use in pregnancy, 108*b*
divalproex sodium
  best evidence of efficacy, 75*b*
  side effects, 78*b*

electroencephalogram (EEG),
    13, 14*f*
eletriptan, 58*b*, 111*b*
emergency room, 1, 164*b*
  chronic migraine, 120
  head injuries, 157
  migraine management, 50*b*,
    54, 56, 57
  migraines and pregnancy, 104,
    106, 110, 111
  rescue plan, 60*b*, 61–62
  severe headaches, 126

encephalitis, 17
epileptic seizures, 13, 31
episodic
    cluster headaches, 145–46, 151
    migraines, 31, 33, 78, 80, 113,
        116–18, 120, 169
    tension-type headaches, 135,
        136*b*, 140*b*
ergotamine, risk for use in
    pregnancy, 108*b*, 109
ergot drugs, 57
erythrocyte sedimentation rate
    (ESR), 114*b*, 137–38
eucalyptus oil, 69
exercise
    children and
        adolescents, 98–99
    physical, as preventive, 86
    tension-type headaches, 139
exertional headaches, 7
exertion-related headaches, 4*b*
eye strain, 32

false message pain, 18
familial hemiplegic migraine
    (FHM), 41*b*
family history, migraines, 31–32
feverfew, 85, 86
fight or flight response, 89–91
Fioricet, 15, 56*b*, 57, 66, 169
Fiorinal, 56*b*, 57
flunarizine, 80
fluoxetine, 78
foods, 27–28, 56, 74, 79, 87–88
fortification spectra, 39*b*
frovatriptan, 58*b*, 75*b*

gabapentin
    migraine preventive, 76*b*

risk for use in pregnancy, 108*b*
    side effects, 78*b*
gastroparesis, 126
gender, migraines by, 25, 25*f*
genetics, migraine, 41–42
genogram, family with
    migraine, 32*f*
giant cell arteritis (GCA), 137,
    138*b*, 140
ginger, 69, 93

Headache Cooperative of New
    England, 172–73
Headache Cooperative of the
    Pacific, 173
headache diary, 47, 49*f*
    case story, 92–93
    chronic migraine patient, 116*f*
    first headache
        appointment, 164*b*
    materials for follow-up
        visits, 168*b*
    parents of children with
        migraines, 96
headaches
    managing by type, *xvi–xvii*
    nerve blocks for, 127–28, 129*b*
    new daily persistent headache
        (NDPH), 139, 140,
        143, 153–55
    phase of migraine, 27*f*
    post-concussive, 158–59
    primary, 2, 4*b*, 4–8
    related to sexual activity, 7–8
    searching for underlying
        medical cause, 10*b*
    secondary, 2, 8–18, 9*b*
    See also primary headaches;
        secondary headaches

Headache: The Journal of Head and Face Pain (journal), 172
head and facial problems, 17
head injuries, 31*b*
  concussion, 157–59
  post-concussive
    syndrome, 159–62
head trauma, risk for chronic
    migraines, 118*b*
health providers. *See*
    communication with
    medical team
heart disease, 125
heat waves, 29, 40
hemicrania continua, 7, 26*b*
  description of, 152*b*
  indomethacin, 7, 138*b*, 145*b*,
    152*b*, 153
  mimic of tension-type
    headache, 138*b*
  trigeminal autonomic
    cephalalgia (TAC), 152–53
hemiplegic migraine, 41*b*, 42
herbal treatments, migraine,
    69–70, 84–86
heroin, headaches, 16
Hippocrates, 27
histamines, 87–88
history, migraine in, 36
holes in vision, scotoma,
    39*b*, 39*f*
homeopathy, 86
hormonal changes, 28*b*
hydrocodone, 60
hydroxyzinc, nausea, 57, 60*b*, 62
hypertension, 12
hyperthyroidism, 51, 117
hypnic headaches, 7
hypnosis, 70, 90, 92
hypothyroidism, 117, 138*b*

ibuprofen, 4, 5, 15, 52
  breastfeeding and, 110, 111*b*
  case story, 92
  headache treatment, 56
  tension-type headaches, 5,
    139, 140*b*
ice cream headache, 28*b*
indomethacin, 99, 138*b*, 145*b*
  anti-inflammatory
    medication, 7, 56*b*, 99
  hemicrania continua, 7, 138*b*,
    145*b*, 152*b*, 153
  paroxysmal hemicrania, 145*b*,
    150, 150*b*
  suppository, 57
infection, 17
inflammation, 11, 37, 38*f*, 114*b*
infusions, hospital treatment,
    131–32, 133*b*
International Classification of
    Headache Disorders (ICHD),
    1, 24, 113, 135
International Headache
    Society, 1, 173
intracranial hypertension
    headaches, 12
iontophoresis, 127
isometheptene/
    dichoralphenazone/
    acetaminophen, 56*b*

juniper, 86

ketamine, hospital
    treatment, 133*b*
ketorolac, 57
kudzu, 86

LactMed, pregnancy and
    lactation, 108

lamotrigine, cluster
  headache, 148
lidocaine
  anesthetic, 128, 133*b*, 152
  hospital treatment, 133*b*
  nerve blocks, 108*b*, 109, 111*b*
  risk for use in pregnancy, 108*b*
life cycle, migraines by gender,
  25, 25*f*
lifestyle strategies, children and
  adolescents, 98*b*
lightheadedness, 40
lisinopril, 76*b*, 79, 81
lithium, cluster headache, 6, 148
low intracranial pressure,
  headaches, 12
lumbar puncture, chronic
  migraine, 12, 114*b*, 119

magnesium, 69, 89, 93, 111*b*,
  112, 133*b*
magnetic resonance imaging
  (MRI), 2
  arteriovenous malformation
    (AVM), 11*f*
  brain, 51
  chronic migraine, 114*b*, 119
  patient undergoing, 3*f*
magnetic stimulation, 131, 132*f*
marijuana, headaches, 16,
  69–70
massage, 86–87, 115
mass lesions, 25, 26*b*, 138*b*
medical conditions, migraine
  associated with, 30–32
medical illness, headaches
  and, 17–18
medical team. *See*
  communication with
  medical team

medical treatment
  acute migraine
    medications, 56*b*
  children and teens, 99–100
  choosing options by attack
    characteristics, 56–59
  fundamentals of, 55–56
  hospital treatment, 133*b*
  infusions and hospital
    treatments, 131–32
  magnetic stimulation, 131, 132*f*
  medications for nausea and
    vomiting, 60*b*
  nerve blocks, 127–28, 129*b*
  nerve stimulation, 129–31
  new forms of
    medication, 126–27
  patients, 53–54, 61–63
  pregnant patients, 106–10
  recurrence and rescue
    options, 59–61
  rescue plans, 60*b*
  tailoring, 54–55
  triptan medications, 58*b*
  See also medical treatment;
    non-medical treatment;
    preventive medication
medication overuse headaches,
  13–16, 31
  case stories, 14–15, 23, 33
  mimic of tension-type
    headache, 138*b*
  risk for chronic migraines, 118*b*
  See also analgesic rebound
    headache
meditation, 70, 91–92
melatonin, 97, 148
meningitis, 17
menstrual periods, 5, 15, 28, 28*b*,
  49*f*, 51, 75*b*, 76*b*, 96–97, 103

menthol, 69, 85
metabolic problems, 17
methylergonovine, unusual
    headaches, 154
metoclopramide
    anti-nausea drug, 45, 60*b*
    breastfeeding and, 111*b*
    movement disorder, 52
    risk for use in pregnancy, 108*b*
metoprolol, best evidence of
    efficacy, 75*b*
MIDAS (Migraine Disability
    Assessment Scale), 47, 48*b*
migraine, 2
    aftermath of attack, 27*f*, 30
    aura, 27*f*, 29
    classification, 31
    clinical stories, 21–23, 32–34
    conditions that mimic, 26*b*
    description of, 24–26
    diagnosing, 32–34
    diagnostic criteria, 24
    disability due to, 45–47
    escape from attack, *xvi*
    family history, 31–32
    features of, 29–30
    gender, 25
    genetics of, 41–42
    goals in managing, 47, 50, 50*b*
    in history, 36
    medical conditions associated
        with, 30–32
    missed work and school, 46*f*
    phases of attack, 27*f*
    prevalence throughout life
        span, 25*f*
    primary headache, 2, 4, 4*b*
    process of, 38*f*
    resources, 171–73

self-assessment checklist, 33*b*
triggers, 26–29
Migraine Action Association, 172
mitochondrial encephalomyopathy,
    lactic acidosis and stroke-like
    episodes (MELAS), 41*b*
monoclonal antibody
    therapies, 127
monogenic causes of migraine,
    41*b*, 42
monosodium glutamate (MSG),
    28*b*, 87–88, 88*b*
muscles
    contraction headache, 136*b*
    relaxation, 70, 105, 158
    tensing of, 89–91, 95
Montefiore Headache Center,
    New York, 45

nadolol, 76*b*
naproxen, breastfeeding and,
    110, 111*b*
naproxen sodium, 51, 56, 56*b*,
    82, 140*b*, 150, 169
naratriptan, 58*b*, 76*b*
narcotics, 23, 33, 123, 145, 165
National Headache
    Foundation, 172
nausea
    childhood migraines
        with, 95–97
    concussion and, 158
    headache diary, 116*f*
    headaches with, 4–5, 10, 15,
        21–23, 35, 62, 125
    medication for, 45, 57, 60*b*,
        69–70, 85, 93
    migraine medication causing,
        53, 55, 61, 126

migraines with, 24, 29, 33*b*,
43–45, 65, 152
pregnancy and, 104, 108, 112
tension-type headache
without, 135, 136*b*
NDPH. *See* new daily persistent
headache (NDPH)
nebivolol, 76*b*
neck problems, 17
nerve blocks, 127–28, 129*b*. *See
also* occipital nerve blockade
nerve stimulation, 129–31, 149
neuralgia, 18
new daily persistent headache
(NDPH), 139, 140, 143
description of, 153*b*
mimic of tension-type
headache, 138*b*
treatment of, 154–55
unusual headache
type, 153–54
nitrites/nitrates, 28*b*, 87–88
noninvasive electrical
stimulation, 130*f*, 131
non-medical treatment
acting on warnings of
impending attack, 66–67
acupressure points, 65, 68*f*
aromatherapy, 69
behavioral medicine
techniques, 70
caffeine, 67–68
case stories, 65–66,
83–84, 92–93
dietary supplements, 89
herbal treatment,
69–70, 84–86
magnesium, 69
manual techniques, 86–87

marijuana, 69–70
meditation and
relaxation, 89–92
nutritional
intervention, 87–88
physical exercise, 86
pregnant patients, 106
nortriptyline, tension-type
headaches, 139, 140*b*
NSAIDs (non-steroidal anti-
inflammatory drugs), 56,
56*b*, 57, 139, 140*b*, 150
nummular headaches, 7
nutraceutical therapy, 85
nutritional intervention, 87–88

obesity, 31*b*, 117, 118*b*
occipital nerve blockade, 109–10,
112, 129*b*
cluster headaches, 148, 149
patient having, 128*f*
post-concussive
headaches, 158
See also nerve blocks
odors, 28*b*
onabotulinumtoxinA
best evidence of efficacy, 75*b*
FDA-approved treatment, 80
patient having injection, 121*f*
preventive therapy, 82,
120–22, 126
ondansetron
breastfeeding and, 111*b*
nausea, 60*b*
risk for use in pregnancy, 108*b*
opioid drugs 16, 60*b*
Organisation for Understanding
Cluster Headache
(OUCH), 173

Osler, William, 69–70
oxycodone, 60, 123
OxyContin, 16
oxygen inhalation, cluster
    headache, 6, 147–48

paresis, migraine, 39*b*, 40
paresthesias, 39*b*
paroxysmal hemicrania
    description of, 150*b*
    indomethacin, 145*b*, 150, 150*b*
    trigeminal autonomic
        cephalalgia (TAC), 150–51
passionflower, 86
peppermint, 86
Percocet, 15, 66, 123
phases of migraine, 27*f*
phobias, chronic migraine, 119
physical exercise, 86, 98–99
pindolol, 76*b*
polygenic causes of
    migraine, 41–42
positron emission tomography
    (PET), 161
post-concussive syndrome
    (PCS), 159–62
    case story, 159–60
    symptoms of post-traumatic
        stress disorder (PTSD), 161*b*
    traumatic brain injury, 160–62
    traumatic brain injury
        symptoms, 160*b*
postdrome
    aftermath of migraine, 30
    phase of migraine, 27*f*
post-traumatic headaches,
    9–10, 138*b*
post-traumatic stress disorder
    (PTSD), 80, 120
    diagnosis of, 159, 162

risk factor for migraine
    "chronification," 118*b*
potassium, 79, 120
prednisone
    cluster headaches, 6
    refractory headaches, 110
pregnancy
    case stories, 104–5, 111–12
    commonly used migraine
        medications by risk
        type, 108*b*
    FDA categories of medication
        risk in, 107*b*
    medication use and
        risks, 106–10
    migraine medications risk for
        use in, 108*b*
    migraines, *xvi*
    phases of migraine
        management, 105–6
    risks of valproate, 79,
        80–81, 109
    triptan drugs and, 108–9
Pregnancy and Lactation
    Labeling Rule, 107
preventive medication, 71
    antidepressants, 77–78
    anti-seizure, 78–79
    benefits and undesired
        effects, 72*t*
    with best evidence of
        efficacy, 75*b*
    beta blockers, 77
    blood pressure
        medications, 79–80
    calcium channel
        blockers, 79–80
    case stories, 73–74, 81–82
    causing regarding
        pregnancy, 80–81

choosing, 71–74
common side effects, 78*b*
cyproheptadine, 80
with less evidence but
    useful, 76*b*
options for, 75–80
overlapping options, 76*f*
See also medical treatment;
    non-medical treatment
primary headaches, 2, 4*b*
cluster headaches, 6–7
migraine, 2, 4
rare conditions, 7–8
tension-type headaches, 4–6
procaine, 128
prochlorperazine, risk for use in
    pregnancy, 108*b*
prodromal symptoms, aura, 66
prodrome, phase of migraine,
    27, 27*f*
progressive muscle relaxation, 70
promethazine
breastfeeding and, 111*b*
nausea, 60*b*
pregnant patients, 112
risk for use in pregnancy,
    108, 108*b*
suppository, 57, 60*b*, 62
propranolol, 51, 74
benefits and undesired
    effects, 72*t*
best evidence of efficacy, 75*b*
breastfeeding and, 110
chronic migraine, 115
risk for use in pregnancy,
    108*b*
side effects, 78*b*
pseudotumor cerebri, 12
psilocybin mushrooms, 16
psychedelics, headaches, 16

Raynaud's phenomenon,
    31, 77, 80
recreational drug use, headaches
    and, 16
recurrence, treatment
    options, 59–61
refractory headaches, 110,
    149, 170
relationships, migraine and, 46*b*
relaxation, meditation and,
    89–92, 105
The Relaxation Response
    (Benson), 90
rescue plans, 55
migraine relief, 60*b*
treatment options, 59–61
resources, 171–73
restless legs syndrome, 120
riboflavin, 89, 110, 111*b*
rizatriptan
case story, 73, 81
for children, 100
moderate-to-severe
    migraine, 58*b*

school, migraine and, 4, 22, 45,
    46*b*, 46*f*, 48*b*, 66, 71
scientific advances,
    understanding migraine, 37
scintillations, aura, 39*b*
scotoma, holes in vision, 39*b*, 39*f*
secondary headaches, 2, 8–9, 9*b*
blood vessels and
    headaches, 10–11
brain malformations, 12
brain tumors, 13
intracranial hypertension
    headaches, 12
low intracranial pressure
    headaches, 12

secondary headaches (*cont.*)
  medical illness, 17–18
  medication overuse
    headaches, 13–16
  neuralgia, 18
  post-traumatic
    headaches, 9–10
  recreational drug use, 16
  seizures, 13
seizures, 13, 31, 72*t*
selective serotonin reuptake
  inhibitor (SSRI), 78
self-assessment checklist,
  diagnosing migraine, 33*b*
self-hypnosis, 70, 92
serotonin-norepinephrine
  reuptake inhibitor
  (SNRI), 78
sexual activity, headaches
  related to, 7–8
short-lasting unilateral
  neuralgiform (SUN)
  headache, 145*b*
  description of, 151*b*
  treatment of, 155
  trigeminal autonomic
    cephalalgia (TAC), 151–52
sinus headache, 21, 32, 33, 44
sleep apnea, 31*b*, 117–18, 118*b*,
  120, 138*b*
sleep disturbances, 28, 31, 120
smoked incense, 16
snoring, 31*b*, 117, 118*b*
social life, migraine and, 46*b*
sodium valproate, infusion
  of, 132
sphenopalatine ganglion
  intranasal infusion for
    blockade of, 129*b*, 129*f*
  stimulation of, 149

spina bifida, valproate, 79
spinal tap, chronic migraine, 12,
  114*b*, 119
status migrainosus, 30
stinging nettle, 86
stomach paralysis,
  gastroparesis, 126
stress response, 89–91
subarachnoid hemorrhage, 11
sumatriptan, 104
  for adolescents, 100
  breastfeeding and, 110, 111*b*
  case stories, 73, 81–82
  cluster headaches, 7, 147
  delivery methods, 51, 52
  headache diary, 116*f*
  injection, 7, 51, 58*b*, 59*f*, 61,
    143–44, 147, 154
  migraine treatment, 33, 43, 122
  moderate-to-severe
    migraine, 58*b*
  nasal powder, 51, 58*b*
  nasal spray, 51, 52, 58*b*, 58*f*,
    100, 126–27
  pregnancy and, 108–9, 111
  tablet, 43, 52, 58*b*, 73, 169
  unusual headaches, 154
SUN. *See* short-lasting unilateral
  neuralgiform (SUN)
  headache
support groups, 100, 172

TACs. *See* trigeminal autonomic
  cephalalgias (TACs)
tardive dyskinesia, 52
temporal arteritis, 137
temporomandibular joint (TMJ)
  disorder, 17, 32, 138*b*
tension-type headache
  (TTH), 2, 135

case stories, 136–37, 140–41
characteristics of, 136*b*
description of, 135–37
mimics of, 137–39, 138*b*
patient-drawn diagram
of, 138*f*
primary, 4*b*, 4–6
treatment of, 139, 140*b*
Teris, pregnancy and
lactation, 108
thyroid disease, 31*b*, 117, 118*b*
thyroid test, 51, 114*b*, 122
Tiger Balm, 69
timolol, best evidence of
efficacy, 75*b*
tizanidine, 76*b*, 108*b*
topiramate, 74
anti-seizure, 78–79
benefits and undesired
effects, 72*t*
best evidence of efficacy,
75*b*, 126
chronic migraine, 120, 123
cluster headache, 148
risk for use in pregnancy,
108*b*, 109
side effects, 78*b*, 79
tension-type headaches,
139, 140*b*
traumatic brain injury (TBI)
post-concussive syndrome
(PCS), 160–62
symptoms in PCS, 160*b*
treatment. *See* medical
treatment; non-medical
treatment
trepanning, 36
trephination, 36
trigeminal autonomic
cephalalgias (TACs), 7, 143

case stories of,
143–44, 154–55
cluster headache, 145–49
hemicrania continua, 152–53
paroxysmal
hemicrania, 150–51
short-lasting unilateral
neuralgiform (SUN)
headache, 151–52
types of, 145*b*
trigeminal neuralgia, 18
triggers
migraine, 26–29
process of migraine, 38*f*
some migraine, 28*b*
triptans, 33, 57, 63, 66
for adolescents and
children, 100
migraine preventives, 76*b*
moderate-to-severe
migraine, 58*b*
in pregnancy, 108–9
risk for use in pregnancy, 108*b*
tyramine, 28*b*, 87

United Council for Neurologic
Subspecialties, 163, 173
US Food and Drug
Administration
(FDA), 57, 59
anti-seizure
medications, 78–79
FDA categories of medication
risk in pregnancy,
107, 107*b*
onabotulinumtoxinA, 121

vagus nerve, stimulation of,
149
valerian root, 86

valproate, 74
anti-seizure, 78–79
benefits and undesired
effects, 72t
best evidence of efficacy, 75b
birth defects, 79, 80–81, 109
chronic migraine, 115
cluster headache, 148
preventive medication, 52
risk for use in pregnancy,
108b, 109
risks in pregnant
women, 80–81
vasculitis, 11
venlafaxine
migraine preventive, 76b, 78
tension-type headaches,
139, 140b
verapamil
benefits and undesired
effects, 72t
cluster headaches, 6, 148
migraine preventive, 76b,
80, 109
risk for use in pregnancy, 109
side effects, 115
vertigo, 29, 30, 40, 158
Vicodin, 16
vitamins, 89, 98, 111b, 126

wavy vision, aura, 38, 39b
websites, resources, 171–73

willow, 86
wine, 74, 87–88, 137
women
birth control pills, 79
chronic headache, 117
cluster headache, 145–47
menstrual periods, 5, 15,
28, 28b, 49f, 51, 75b, 76b,
96–97, 103
migraines in, 4–5, 24–25,
25f
pregnancy, 79, 80–81,
103, 105–9
See also pregnancy
work, migraine and, 46b
World Health Organization
(WHO), xv, 24

zigzag lines, migraine aura, 39b,
39f, 40
zolmitriptan
breastfeeding and, 110, 111b
migraine preventive, 76b
moderate-to-severe
migraine, 58b
nasal spray, 58b, 126
pregnancy and, 108
zonisamide
migraine preventive, 76b
risk for use in pregnancy,
108b
side effects, 78b